Breaking The Silence

The Stigma of Mental Illness

Polly Fielding

Copyright © 2015 Polly Fielding
All rights reserved.

ISBN-13: 978-1515016236
ISBN-10: 1515016234

All profits from this book will be donated to the UK charity SANE which is fighting to eradicate mental health stigma

All rights reserved, no part of this publication may be reproduced by any means, electronic, mechanical photocopying, documentary, film or in any other format without prior written permission of the author

Copyright for each story is held by its author

Cover art by Polly Fielding

Other Books by Polly Fielding

And This Is My Adopted Daughter

A Mind To Be Free

Crossing The Borderline

Letting Go

Missing Factor (A personal experience of haemophilia)

Going In Seine

Nurturing Compassion

Moments Of Mindfulness

Time For Mindfulness

Mindfulness For The 5:2 Diet

The 5:2 Diet Made eZy

The 5:2 Vegetarian Diet Made eZy

Single Serving Recipes To Soothe Arthritis

Single Serving Vegetarian Recipes To Soothe Arthritis

Delicious Vegetarian Diabetic Meals For One

Vegetarian Recipes For One To Lower Blood Pressure

A Veritable Smorgasbord

www.pollyfielding.com

DEDICATION

To everyone who contributed to 'Breaking The Silence' and to all who experience the painful, damaging stigma that surrounds mental illness.

Some names have been changed to protect identities and respect confidentiality

CONTENTS

Foreword	7
Introduction	9
Lizzie's Story	15
Valerie's Story	19
Timothy's Story	29
Penny's Story	41
Maisie's Story	55
Daniel's Story	61
Emma''s Story	65
Maria's Story	81
Colin's Story	93
Amy Jean's Story	101
Lauren's Story	123
Kil's Story	129
Bridget's Story	137
Alma's Story	143
Simon's Story	161
Some Useful Online Resources	181

Breaking The Silence

Foreword

You may feel 'tumble-dried' by the whirlwind of human existence so powerfully shared in this book. In equal measure it has been an emotional, upsetting, rewarding and hopeful experience to read so many people's journeys with their mental health.

I'll correct that, as this is actually more about each author's journey with life more broadly, with mental health as a core aspect.

The impact of each author's mental health issues, treatment and support (or the lack of it), and then the pure injustice of stigma and discrimination is laid bare on these pages.

The far reaching consequences of having to deal with stigma are sitting more subtly between the lines of some stories but in others these are more starkly set out; the loss of friendships, isolation from your own family, the loss of jobs, the withdrawal of job offers and college/training places, the breakdown of relationships, the lack of hope for recovery, the loss of self-esteem, self-confidence and self-worth, the powerful sense of being made to feel "other" and the threat to life itself.

Being willing to publically share such deeply personal, and often very traumatic, experiences with us readers must have taken a great deal of energy, strength and courage.

By doing so in this book, each person who has told their story will be passing on that energy, strength and courage to others as well as helping to inform and transform public understanding and attitudes.

For which, I can't thank each author enough.

Polly's own determination and passion seem to have worked like a magical magnet to bring this collection of people together to write their stories. I'm very honoured and privileged to have been asked to read this book. Thousands of us with experience of mental health problems are working together to tackle mental health stigma and discrimination.

I hope this book inspires you to do the same.

Sue Baker, Director, Time to Change

Introduction

Silence is powerful.

Silently watching the glowing, changing colours of a setting sun is uplifting and enriching. Mindful self-reflection is nourishing. Being in a hushed auditorium during a virtuoso performance is a shared, inspiring experience.

But the silence of family, friends and colleagues when I had a complete mental breakdown had an oppressive, alienating feel to it.

When I was admitted to a psychiatric hospital and took early retirement from teaching, only the standard written acknowledgement from the Department for Education marked the end of a long career. There was no customary leaving present from the staff of the school where I had taught for the previous eight years, no letter of thanks from the Head, no flowers, not even a get well card…

It was as though I'd never existed in the place where I'd felt so valued by parents and children. I felt completely worthless, undeserving, ashamed and totally rejected.

And relatives' uncomfortable silent response, to my

eight months' stay in an acute ward, forced me to appear outwardly 'normal' whilst withdrawing inwardly even further into the painful desolation of shame, guilt, frustration and self-directed anger.

Sadly, mine is not an isolated case. I'm one of many.

With formerly taboo topics like 'sex' and 'cancer' now being discussed freely, wouldn't you think that there'd be a greater degree of openness and a genuine understanding of the mental health problems suffered by so many of us in society?

But whilst physical ailments generally evoke a positive, sympathetic response from others, such is the stigma around mental health issues that it continues to be viewed with a massive dose of fear, ignorance and denial.

This destructive, wide-spread attitude in society has a devastating effect on sufferers, making it far harder for them to access treatment or even to ask for help in the first place. It encourages secrecy amongst employees about any emotional difficulties for fear of losing their jobs.

And despite claiming otherwise, governments continue to give low priority status to much-needed mental health services, when it actually comes down to financing resources for them. Meanwhile, people with mental illnesses on long waiting lists are taking their lives before the treatment they so urgently need becomes available.

I've listened to caring mental health professionals talk about how, tasked with constantly assessing the risk clients pose to themselves, they are becoming increasingly disillusioned about ever being allowed to deliver specific treatments to them. The money simply isn't there for them to do the jobs they've spent years training to do. They too feel devalued.

Unfortunately, not every health professional, even within the Mental Health System, really understands the nature of mental illness and an approach which sends a clear message to service users that they are 'wasting precious NHS resources' can be incredibly damaging.

I know what it's like to feel like a pariah in society and I was tired of feeling out of control. I became desperate to show I was worth the therapies finally allowed me. So I endured the numerous assessments deemed necessary to prove, beyond all reasonable doubt, that treating me would be cost-effective in the long term.

Without the positive coping mechanisms to deal with my 'Borderline Personality Disorder' that Mindfulness Based Cognitive Therapy and Dialectical Behaviour Therapy gave me, I could not have survived.

Since I joined Twitter I've become more aware of others' lack of accessibility to mental health services and the huge gap in provision of resources which, at best, results in massive emotional pain for sufferers and, at worst, contributes to suicides. I am also infuriated by comments on social networks which reflect the ignorance of mental illness such as, 'Why doesn't he hurry up and jump?' - reference to a distressed man who was causing a traffic jam by threatening to throw himself off a bridge, over the M61.

Some, who know first-hand what it is like to live with the daily torment of mental illness, find creative ways to express their pain to the rest of the world. A glance through the history of the arts reveals numerous famous musicians, writers and artists who were mentally ill yet who left an important legacy. Robert Schumann, Amy Winehouse, Sylvia Plath, Edvard Munch, to name a few... all had severe mental health problems.

Frustrated with the extent of the stigma that surrounds mental illness, I decided to tap into the creativity of others with experience of mental health problems. Enthusiastically, I started looking for people on Twitter, willing to be a part of my project; but after a few weeks I became discouraged; perhaps it was simply too much to ask people to trust me with such sensitive material.

At that point that I received Lizzie's superbly written story which moved me to tears; it was the extra bit of motivation I needed. I owed it to her, at least, to continue.

Over the next couple of months fourteen powerfully written accounts followed, each one a unique and intensely moving expression of their suffering.

I was unprepared for how strongly I would be affected by them. I could identify a bit too closely with a lot of their suffering. I also began to worry about the effect that delving into the past and expressing such immense emotional pain was having on the writers, particularly those who have not yet accessed treatment specific for their needs.

It was with relief that I read that, although painful, writing their stories was cathartic for many, inspiring some of them to begin writing their own books. Without exception, they wanted others to hear their voices, to play their part in dispelling stigma by vividly showing people what it's actually like to live with mental illness. And the negative impact of people's reactions to their illness needs to be heard.

I am so grateful to all the contributors within these

pages for their brave and compellingly-written stories. Together we will cut through the destructive silence.

Lizzie's Story

I managed to keep myself going for my child and teenage years and it wasn't until my early twenties that I began to lose my grip on pretending to be ok. I was abused from a young age and I hid it from everyone until I was severely depressed with suicidal thoughts and could no longer leave the house without blacking out from anxiety attacks. My boyfriend at the time couldn't comprehend the darkness I was in and, although we had been together for five years, he could no longer cope with me and we ended our relationship. I will never forget him crying, saying he couldn't be with me wondering if one day he'd come home and find me dead; the impact of someone leaving me for the thing I had no control over hurt me more than anything I had been through and the fact that he didn't understand how he could help was agony. It is because of this that I find it hard to imagine ever being able to have a relationship again, or whether a relationship where I hide my mental illness is the only option.

It was around this time that I was signed off work and not long after, I was admitted into the psychiatric unit for my own safety. My friends at the time never understood mental illness, it was foreign to them. I lost count of the amount of times I was told to sleep it off or do exercise to break my mood, but to them I was a project to fix. After they realised I couldn't be fixed with pep talks and exercise they lost interest and drifted away from me as though I was a lost cause or for fear they would catch something from me. My friends' lack of empathy made me feel even more isolated than I could have ever imagined. Having no safety net left I plummeted and it took years to regain the confidence to trust people or believe in people again.

It was this similar attitude to mental illness that meant I was forced to leave my job a few years later. Occupational Health's words were along the lines of "There are no longer any more reasonable adjustments we can make to keep you at work and make you a reliable member of the team" - something that cut through me as even on my worst days I had dragged myself into work but, yes, I had a fair amount of time off. However, at the age of twenty-six to be told that you are no longer an asset felt like no one in the world believed I could get better. The reasonable adjustments that had been made included forcing me to leave the job I loved because the manager used to shout at me making me cry in full view of everyone and I was pushed into an office where I spent 80% of my day photocopying, on my own in a hot cubby hole where I would sob my heart out as I photocopied mounds of paper the same height as me. At this point, I no longer cared about anything as I was living with flashbacks, severe depression and crippling anxiety that ruled my life and my ability to live. I felt betrayed by everyone and that I had nothing left to live for; then my second admission to the psychiatric unit happened.

For now I have a more positive present; after the second admission to the psychiatric unit I decided to start a college course and get a degree that would help me to campaign for Mental Health issues and better awareness. I start university in September and my abuser is now in prison. But I do feel that if people were more understanding or took the time to listen to me rather than write me off then I could have perhaps stayed out of the psychiatric unit and had my care managed in the community. If people hadn't been scared of the answers I may have given them then they would have hung around and helped, walking alongside me through the darkness. It's not so much about what you say but it's the times you're there on the sofa not saying a word, just being there is more than enough. I would much rather explain to someone how mental illness affects me than for people to not understand and hide. The attitudes I have been shown have stopped me from trusting new people and I often hide the truth as to why I might not be around for a few days in fear of losing friends. Hopefully, this is something I can work on in the future by listening to myself and creating more awareness.

Valerie's Story

I am Valerie and I will give you my story in two parts. The first part will tell you about my background, how I came into contact with the Mental Health Services and how I live my life today. The second will tell you about the treatments I have had and the impact they had on me.

I grew up in Ireland and am the youngest of three girls. Home life was difficult but I was made to believe that I was very fortunate to have the life I had. My father was a very heavy drinker but also a very hard worker. My mother worked as a dressmaker, working about twelve hours a day. Having money was very important to both of them. They both wanted the best for their children.

I was a very sensitive child and I was beaten very severely if I did anything wrong. One of the worst things that I could do was look for attention or ask for help. At school I did very well because achieving was one way that I could get attention from my parents, whom I was very eager to please. There was a lot of responsibility put on me at a very young age and from nine years old I used to have to go to town and do the weekly shopping.

During these shopping trips I started going into

amusement arcades. It was there that I befriended the manager who was probably about fifty. He was very kind and caring to me and gave me loads of attention. However, as time went on, sexual abuse started to occur. I didn't stop him because he was so kind and nice to me. I felt very guilty because even though I was only nine, I knew it was wrong. This abuse continued until I was about fourteen. I never told anyone about it until I went into therapy because I always felt I was to blame having allowed him to do these things to me.

I went to University and gained two degrees but I had zero self belief. I started work as a teacher but I hated it and I then got a job in the Civil Service. All the time I was desperate to please my mother. I had a relationship that lasted for about four years but my mother disapproved of him.

Eventually I left him and met a man whom my mother adored and I eventually married. It was the first time in my life that I had gained her approval.

Married life was good but I did everything to please my husband. I had two children and on the outside everything looked OK. A turning point for me came about when I wanted a third child and my husband refused to have one. I felt very resentful. During this time, both my parents died and one of my sisters was diagnosed with breast cancer. I felt totally overwhelmed but did not ask for help because I felt it was a sign of weakness. I coped by drinking alcohol. Up to this point in my life I had rarely drunk.

About twelve years ago I had a major breakdown and this is how I first came into contact with the mental health services. I just wanted to die and I very firmly believed that my children would be better off without me. I made a number of very serious attempts to kill myself and it is a miracle that I survived. I was admitted to the DOP (Department of Psychiatry) in Southampton and was diagnosed with very serious clinical depression. I battled on for many years and the only treatment I received was medication, which I now believe had little or no beneficial effect.

Some years later I received psychological therapy, which I will tell you about in the second part of my story and which totally transformed my life.

So how I am today?

For the first time in my life I feel totally at ease with myself. I spent most of my life hating myself, believing that I was evil. Today I feel good about myself.

At the start of my treatment I had one goal and that was to just want to survive. I never dreamed that I could ever have a life truly worth living, but this is what I have today. I no longer have major crises in my life on a day to day basis. In the past, a crisis to me was getting on a wrong bus. I still have the stresses of ordinary everyday life, going to work, running a home and dealing with stroppy teenagers, but the difference now is that I can cope. When something new arises, I stand back for half a second and ask myself what I can do in this situation. I now have a whole range of skills to choose from to help me deal with everyday life.

I now feel I have great freedom because I have choice. I don't have to follow my mind all the time. Emotions had taken over my life, but now I feel in control. I now accept the life I have and I am enjoying it. I spent years trying to change my husband and others around me, but never succeeded. This is something that I now don't even attempt and amazingly their response to me and the way they treat me has changed. I no longer go around chasing good feelings and avoiding bad ones, instead I am leading a full and meaningful life. Most of the time I now live my life in the present and I appreciate it in its fullness. The past is nothing more than memories and the future is just thoughts and images. I have made many changes to my life; I left my job as a civil servant which I had worked in for twenty-seven years. I was a square peg in a round hole.

Today I work as a senior Peer Support Worker in an acute Mental Health ward. I come home from work each day feeling I have made a difference.

I will conclude by saying that my life today is truly worth living and in the second part of my story I will tell you how I got there.

My Story - Part Two

The question is how did I get to the place I am in today?

As I said, for many years the only treatment I received was medication and loads of sympathy which had very little beneficial effect on me. I feel being given the label of clinically depressed took away any responsibility from me for trying to do anything to improve my situation.

I was then offered counselling, which was helpful in that there was someone truly listening to me and empathizing. This for me was really nice and I really liked going there. However, the problem was it was not changing anything and in many ways, it was keeping the depression going because I was getting loads of sympathy. I was also given ECT (Electrical Convulsive Therapy), which blanked things in the short term but did not improve things in the long term. It also severely affected my memory, which I don't think has ever fully come back.

Some years later I was offered CBT (Cognitive Behaviour Therapy) and this did bring about some very positive changes in my life. This was the first time in my life that I realised just how influential thoughts are in the way they make us feel. Up until this point I had never questioned my thoughts, I thought they were facts. Unfortunately the therapy only lasted six months because the therapist was taking up another post.

Following the therapy I coped very well for about eighteen months and, in fact, I coped so well I decided to go for a change of career, but was prevented from doing so at the last minute because of my recorded mental health problems. I thought I could cope with this major disappointment but found I could not accept the situation.

This led me to go back to my old ways of coping.

In 2011 I had four admissions to psychiatric hospitals and was sectioned three times. Luckily I was offered DBT (Dialectical Behaviour Therapy) following the first admission. My journey through

DBT was a very difficult one. Through my work with CAST (Consultancy And Support Team – a service-user involvement group for Southern Health Foundation Trust), I came into contact with people who had benefited from DBT. From what they told me, it appeared to have changed their lives. I believed that DBT would change my life too and that the therapist would somehow magically make it happen. This meant that I myself came to the therapy with what I thought was a very positive attitude and a strong commitment. However the challenge it presented was much greater that I expected.

I spent the first six months resisting DBT and fighting with the therapist, saying things such as "Why do I have to this, nobody else does", and "I can't use these skills - they are a load of rubbish." My commitment to DBT was questioned by the therapist on several occasions and I was up in arms about this because I always attended the sessions and did my homework. The therapist's response was that DBT is like learning to swim. You can pack your bag, get in your car and drive to the pool but not actually get in the pool. I was not fully engaging with the process. I was turning up, but not actively participating

I had numerous falling outs with the therapist. I thought she was very hard on me and privately I called her all the names under the sun. Despite this, I always went back the next week because, even though the therapy was very confrontational and challenging, it was clear to me she had real genuineness and warmth. She always said to me that she practiced what she preached and I could see this was true from the examples she used from her own life where she used DBT skills regularly.

She certainly was very mindful throughout the sessions even though at the time I wished she would 'tune out' sometimes.

Her commitment to me was unwavering throughout, despite my own commitment being sometimes less than it should have been.

Our battles continued until one day the penny finally dropped for me. In the days before this session I had once again resorted to destructive coping mechanisms to deal with an everyday stress. I rang her up and told her I was not going to attend the session that day because I felt so bad and I was incapable of getting the bus to the session. She told me that now was the time to attend and to get a taxi there.

On the telephone she appeared very compassionate and nurturing and convinced me that I should go after all. Once there, however, all hell broke loose and I was forced to face the reality of the situation and this was very painful indeed. It was pointed out to me that I was letting my teenage children down by my willfulness.

For me this was a very hot spot. I attempted to leave the session when faced with this pain but she pointed out I was running away again. I went home in a very bad way but later that day listened to the recording of the session and accepted the reality that was being explained there. I made a new commitment to myself that day, that DBT was going to be the most important thing in my life – everything else, including children, job etc. would have to come second.

I practiced and practiced the skills even when I really didn't want to and after five or six weeks I found myself using the skills without even realising it. Over the next few months my life gradually became easier as the skills became more ingrained and I applied them more easily to everyday life.

Now that I have finished my therapy I regularly play back the recordings of my old therapy sessions. I also act as my own therapist. I have a weekly session with myself. I validate myself, and regularly give myself a pat on the back. I do chain analysis on stressful situations and see if I could have handled them any differently. I think the ultimate goal in therapy is to train the client to be their own therapist.

I will conclude by saying that stigma has probably been the biggest factor which held back my recovery. My work colleagues shunned me and there was often silence when I came into a room. I lost many so-called friends when they became aware that I had tried to end my life. My family don't like me talking about my mental health.

Today I am an open book about my difficulties because I feel "Why shouldn't I? I haven't committed a crime." Being open has helped me a great deal and I also feel it is breaking down stigma.

Timothy's Story

I was, you could say, a problem child growing up. I acted out. I didn't get along well with others. I did inappropriate things. This started back as early as kindergarten. I threw toys. I had temper tantrums. I dropped to the floor to look up the girls' skirts. I even cut off a girl's ponytail. The ponytail incident is what led my parents to take me to a psychiatrist. The doctor diagnosed me as having Attention Deficit Disorder and I was prescribed Ritalin. I had the same reaction any six-year-old would towards taking pills; I did not want to be taking this stuff. I did the trick to beat the "open your mouth so I can see you took the pill" test: I faked putting the pill in my mouth, then quickly pocketed it during the water drinking and the school nurse was none the wiser.

Things at home were not easy, though. I had a physically, verbally, and emotionally abusive father. He did all the old-fashioned punishments. He spanked me. He yelled at me. He made me sit in the corner for hours at a time. He made me wash my mouth out with soap. He denied me privileges. He sent me to bed early. These were the things that led me down my path in life. Sure my mom tried her best against my dad, but my dad had the final say.

One of the biggest emotional hits in my early years was the loss of my childhood best friend when I was seven years old. We grew up together, since my birth. She was less than a year older than me, but her first word ever was when she first saw me. It was "mine." We did everything together. She had a brain tumor since birth but, despite her fighting and successes, she unfortunately succumbed to the cancer. I will say she got her Make-A-Wish trip to Disney World and had a wonderful time before her death, all of which amazed me, and I found it brave that she went on the then new Tower of Terror, way before I had the nerve enough to ride it. I was told she was getting better at first, I still don't know how true that was.

The pressure of her death and my dad's punishment led to me developing a new disorder: Dissociative Identity Disorder, multiple personalities. My first alter was intended to protect me from the impact of my dad's punishments. I sat in the corner too many times. This punishment was an advanced form of "have you learned your lesson?" but his punishments were longer than necessary.

I remember one time, I don't know when in the timeline of my history, but my dad made me sit in the corner for almost eight hours or so. My mom had enough and brought him outside to say things you don't say when your kid's in the room. I remember the yelling, but I was a good boy and stayed in the corner. My mom came into the house, packed things, and took me to a relative's. Three days later my dad came to us, begging for another chance and my mom forgave him. This was what caused my first fracture. I had, of course, imagined I was in a happy place outside of the corner, and I developed The Protector. Whenever dad abused me, The Protector took over and dealt with it, making me feel better and handling the situation until he felt he had resolved the problem. DID is a mental illness which some people don't believe in. They think that it's a put on or a joke or a game or just a person messing around with others. It is very real. It's not a conscious way to act out to avoid blame for something; alters do act this way and should not cause trouble to be blamed on the core personality, but unfortunately this is not the case.

When I was eight, I received the sacrament of Communion. My dad arranged a big party, and relatives came that I didn't even know I had, and still don't. The day after, he asked my mom for a divorce. This was the start of the development of The Aggressor. I was angry at my dad, but also blamed myself. "What if I were a good boy, he wouldn't have left?" Every child whose parents get divorced instinctually feels that the divorce is their fault. Slowly The Aggressor grew more powerful.

I went through ups and downs over the next few years, acting out worse and transitioning back and forth with The Protector and the still developing Aggressor. My parent's joint custody agreement led to me having problems with both of them. I, of course, had anger towards them, blaming each for the divorce. I, of course, had those "I never want to see you again" comments to my dad, who, when I was thirteen years old, replied, "That can be arranged." The situation was that when my dad brought me home to my mom one weekend, he had given the usually idle threat of "clean your room or I'm throwing everything out." Well, he meant it. Watching all my things getting thrown out, then my mother screaming at my father not to throw it out, was what finally solidified The Aggressor. I don't remember much else because I had dissociated, but I did get my possessions. I didn't hear from my dad for almost two years. I of course blamed myself and him for this. I was bullied on suspicions of being gay, which I am not. I got so frustrated I gave in and let The Aggressor be in charge for almost all of my 7th and 8th grade years, to seem tough. Unfortunately, The Aggressor got me in a lot of trouble. The vice principal hated The Aggressor and gave him a seriously hard time.

The Aggressor, however, did not like the fact that he was bullied. Over the course of two years, The Aggressor attempted suicide at least seventeen times, including jumping off the roof, jumping from other high places, trying to drown in a bathtub and even toilet bowl, electrocution attempts, doing physical harm such as cuts, stab wounds, and an attempt to set fire upon us, drinking chemical substances, hanging, and putting a plastic shopping bag on our head. Fortunately none of these attempts succeeded or did severe damage, but they also didn't make the pain go away. To go to school, five days a week, to be laughed at, called names, have things thrown at us, locked in places like lockers and the gym locker room, to be goaded into acts that gave detention, be tripped, knocked over and around, to be beaten up at least three times a week, and have no one to talk to about this; it's really the worst thing imaginable. And my heart now goes out to the kids who are cyber bullied, which wasn't a thing when I was in school. Kids who do absolutely nothing and are treated like garbage, just because they are smart, or mentally ill, or homosexual, or appear a little different or are on medications. These kids are no different from any other kid. We are all human beings, so why are some kids treated like this? Bullying is wrong, and parents, teachers and other school staff should do something about this. My only consolation is that cyber bullies are now easier to catch than regular bullies and bullying can now be held against a student, even if they are off of school grounds.

Due to bullying on the school bus, The Aggressor said the worst four letter word you can say on a school bus: bomb. This nearly got me expelled, but also weakened the power The Aggressor had on me.

I eventually was able to reconcile with my father, who had gotten a job offer in Texas and took it. Since then I see my father once or twice a year.

After graduation, I spent the summer before high school home alone. I really remember very little of it, almost constantly with The Aggressor in control. The day before my first day of high school, The Aggressor sealed my cat in a QVC cardboard box. The cat swallowed a packing peanut and choked to death. The Aggressor was unprepared for this and retreated away. I then switched to The Protector, who took control of my body for five months, starting with a month long stay on a mental unit. I was then diagnosed as having bipolar disorder rather than ADD, and my medications were switched to reflect that. All of those years I was on medications for an illness I didn't really have. Living with bipolar disorder is what made me want to commit suicide, to be socially awkward, to act out, and to cause all the trouble I was in. I was on a stimulant, which was the absolute worst thing for someone such as myself. I was put on a new cocktail of medications. I hated taking one pill three times a day, now taking six pills a day, and steadily increasing.

In high school, I was accepted into a special education program for those with mental illnesses. Of course, I hated it at first. What kid wants to be placed in a special ed program? The cool kids would think I was stupid. I was embarrassed. But in and out of the program I made many new friends, and once my life had gotten better, The Protector also retreated, giving me full control. With the help of psychiatrists and therapists, I was eventually able to integrate my alters.

My dad surprised me again by marrying without giving me any warning, to a woman who I have never liked. I was, of course, pissed, but I tried to not let that get to me.

I had been a lazy high school student, frequently skipping my mainstream classes with students outside the program. This all changed when my grandmother passed away. We had been very close, and we had a great understanding of each other. We were both slightly crazy and had a lot of time together. Her wake is what caused another alter to

form, The Trickster. In all honesty, The Trickster

was more behaved than my other alters. It also dove me deep into depression. It was not originally The Trickster, but that is what it grew to be. There, a mistake on my grandmother's make-up, if had not been such a sad situation, would have made me laugh so hard, and others find the story funny, too. This spawned The Trickster, who was in charge of my body for almost a year, getting me into trouble. Finally, it got to the point where I skipped every class, staying in the detention room all day. They placed me in all special education classes, from which I blossomed and aced my classes. I unfortunately came down with a crash. I made a superficial cut on my neck and was placed in a mental hospital for two weeks. During the stay, The Trickster decided he had had enough and integrated. When I returned to school, I had developed the paranoia that people only hung around me because I always made a spectacle out of myself in front of the cool kids and withdrew a good deal, including avoiding people in school up until my graduation.

I attended college for three years. My attendance records were a bit spotty and my grades weren't always the greatest, but I made friends, people who didn't know about the cat, or my DID, or paranoia, or the special program in high school, or the evil vice principal in school. It was a fresh start… aside from taking my meds. I was always embarrassed to pop pills during the course of the day. People would think I was a freak or something. So I often hid my pills in my underwear drawer and often skipped them. This made falling asleep highly difficult, and on top of that I also developed a caffeine addiction. I had very little sleep, annoying my roommate with the lights constantly on, and when I really felt tired when wanting to do something, I popped caffeine pills or other caffeine products sold in the campus bookstore. This got so bad that my addiction led to me being up all night and sleeping during class. This led to many problems, including bad grades. These cost me my funds of attending college and I had to leave. I also developed a seizure disorder due to the balance of my medications and caffeine and I was put on more medications, which made me have to take my medications as I had a series of seizures, which really worried my teachers, my classmates, and my roommates. I also underwent the worst betrayal anyone can ever go through. I had a male friend who was gay. I constantly rejected his advances on me, and when I blew up and made several homosexual slurs, he turned it around and raped me. I got a scar an inch over my right eye. I also didn't want to say anything because I was so embarrassed, I felt like it was my fault and that I deserved it, and still wanted to protect the identity of him, and never filed a report. It constantly haunts me, but I think of the scar as a sign of strength and survival, to remember I got through that and could get through anything. Generally, people don't quite realize that men don't get raped and that rape is only men sexually abusing women, but men can be raped by other men, and the emotions are just the same. I find it often difficult to have physical contact with other men, out of the fear of being taken advantage of again. It may seem to be paranoia, but many rape victims feel the same way.

When I was twenty-one, I started to drink alcohol, which is typical for people that age. This, balanced with the medications and caffeine, became a problem. I did overcome my caffeine addiction, but I still do drink coffee, soda, and occasionally an energy drink, but it is not an addiction like it used to be. The alcohol wasn't a real problem at first. I had a job that I was comfortable with, but due to my seizures, I became too much of a liability (which they never said, but we all know that's what it was) and was let go from the job. I started going to the deli up the street and getting several cans of beer a day, and drank alcohol still around the house, including rubbing alcohol and cooking wine, as well as the heavy wines and vodka. It took time, until I realized I was an alcoholic and that my medications and alcohol were causing a huge problem. I have remained sober since the realization of my alcoholic condition. It's still difficult to get over. Simple things are tempting. Hand sanitizers are a huge draw. The smell of it just makes me want to open the bottle and drink it. And Listerine is a huge craving. So many times I just want to swallow it rather than gargle.

I also felt suicidal thoughts recently, seeking the help of inpatient mental hospital stays and an outpatient program following the stays. The leading into the stay was a toxic home environment that was causing me to again wish to commit suicide to end my pain in my house that I just couldn't stand. Both times, I voluntarily admitted myself because I had the moment of clarity, realizing that my life wasn't working the way it was going, the way it was, and a change had to be made. This same feeling occurred when I realized I was an alcoholic.

I have come to the point where I want to be an advocate. I wish to tell my stories and knowledge to those who don't properly understand mental illnesses and eliminate the stigmas behind them, and to offer help to those living with a mental illness to let them know that they are not alone. Life with mental illnesses is difficult, but it can be overcome.

Breaking The Silence

Penny's Story

I remember it so clearly, watching my baby brother being held by our nanny, I was furious, incandescent with rage and I had no idea why. Not really, until the other day when I watched Kate Silverton describe how she saw her daughter's eyes glaze over when she described how she had not been so attentive to her once her second baby was born and how her daughter's behaviour was so bad. Fortunately for her daughter, Kate has the courage and desire to change it for her... that didn't happen for me and my behaviour got totally out of control. I was one year and two weeks old and full of rage.

Things had started before then. I have always wondered what happened to me, it's like my soul has split off and is watching a regular internal crash that it cannot seem to stop; it's the strangest feeling and I have had it all my life. I began to do the research and ask the questions, much to my family's annoyance. They started telling me to stop going on about the past, to stop going on and on about it all, "Just get on with your life Penny"... The trouble was, I couldn't and I needed answers.

I was standing in my kitchen in 2005 when my step-mother, who had been both verbally and physically abusive to me from the age of four and a half to twelve years old, told me that my mother was the first woman to go on a camel in the 60's. When I asked my mother about it she was very sheepish and finally admitted she went on a cruise for six weeks with my father, who had insisted she went with him, when I was four months old. They left me with her step-mother, whom she absolutely hated and who, I have since learnt, had severe post-natal depression due to just having to give a baby daughter away because she could not look after her. My mother went on to say that I was a bit grubby when they picked me up, but she had no choice as nobody else could help and they paid her well... I was utterly stunned. And so it began, the horror of the first year of my life.

I was born in 1960 to an eighteen year old woman and a thirty-eight year old man... she was a waitress and he was her boss. I was not planned and they got married because of me (which I found out when I was fifteen and put the dates together). This answered another question for me: Why had I always felt like the outsider, not 'part of'? It was all very odd. I was with my mother for the first month of my life, although she tells me she was worked off her feet closing down the hotel and moving to Gatwick airport to do the full catering from our flight kitchen. When I asked her where I was she said, "Beside me in a cot..."

At one month old I was given to a Nanny, who my aunt tells me was so unkind to me, she reported it to my parents and they sacked her and then for a little while my aunt had me. She tells me, in a rather degrading way, that I was so precious I was not even allowed on a bus, that they had to take taxis everywhere.

At four months old I was left with Eve, my mother's stepmother and then, when they got back, my grandma (my absolute saviour) had me for a little while, before Nanny Edna came, when I was nine and a half months old. At one and a half years old, my brother is born and that's it, I have gone somewhere else, terrified and very alone. I couldn't bear to see him taken care of by Edna, held and cuddled, and I was supposed to be over that now. But it hadn't ever happened for me and deep down inside my bones, every cell of my body, I know it.

I used to push his pram to the end of the garden and call him bad boy. I did many things to try and get rid of him because I hated him and there was nobody there to help me with it. I now know it was not that I was bad; it was that my feelings were normal and they didn't help me. My mother always bragged about how she had to work eighteen hour days when she was pregnant with him; it wasn't until a lot later I suddenly thought, so where was I? As the pieces of my history slowly came together and why I feel so horrendous inside, it caused me to almost completely break down.

My mother told me I was a very clingy child, apparently people used to comment on it; that I would sit on her lap and rub her petticoat, or sit on the floor next to her and rub it under her skirt. She told me that I would go to their bed at 4am, and snuggle up. How clever was I. They left for work at 5am. I needed some love and if the only way I was going to get it was to get up at 4am, then so be it... I am both heartbroken and deeply impressed as I write and remember this.

I obviously felt close to them on some level, and I know on a deep spiritual level I was. On a good day, they both really got me and I felt they liked me as me and celebrated me as me, which makes it all so much more painful.

I've been told that, at three and a half, I danced on our dining room table and when my aunt said to my father, "Get her off the table", his reply was, "She'll get off when she's finished."...Oh, how I love that story! I love the story of hiding my youngest brother from the doctor because, apparently, I hated injections and when the doctor came I didn't want him to hurt him, so I hid him in my dolls cot! He has no real connection for me, but I loved him so much. I was very jealous of my other brother, that is very sad.

When I was three and a half, the next brother was two and a half and my baby brother was one and a half; all being looked after by one nanny and other staff...our mother left. According to my uncle, I was screaming so loudly he will never ever forget the scream. She left our Christmas presents on the doorstep and, apparently, my father told her not to see us for a while to help us get over it...it was the opposite for me.

We moved house soon after this. I would be in my father's bed a lot. Then he moved a young woman in and I was not allowed in there any more; she was nineteen and he was now forty-three, a very powerful man at Gatwick Airport. She absolutely hated me and would humiliate me, hit me, shove soap in my mouth and ask me who the hell do I think I am. I was distraught. I slowly slipped away...

I used to talk to my grandma, tell her how sad and lonely I was, how I hated my life... the light was very slowly going out in my world and my behaviour was getting more and more erratic. I cut my hair off at five years old, left it up and down the corridor. My stepmother hated my father brushing my hair and would snarl at me from behind the wings of her chair... she terrified me and so I stopped it and cut it off, hoping she would like me now and stop hurting me. I stopped ballet and singing because she humiliated me so much... my dream of being a dancer and actress slipped away because I felt so utterly shit about myself and that I was so awful.

I was sexually abused by a member of staff by the time I was seven years old. I believe this set me up for a life of mental torment.

My stepmother left when I was twelve. We were back in touch with our mother who was not really around and did not understand my needs. She was unreliable and nobody, apart from me, wanted her to visit. She worked very hard and always said it was her work that kept her away. When I saw her wardrobe one day, stuffed with handbags, beautiful dresses and handbags, I was heartbroken.

I have never really recovered from all the distress of this early life. Self- harming, addiction, shoplifting, abusive relationships with friends and lovers and a life of huge highs and lows has left me in a very lonely life. Nobody would ever have known it; I did so well at covering it up.

I have a wonderful son who, to be honest, has been my saviour; without him I seriously do not know if I would be alive. I got sober when I realised my life was affecting him and I have tried, to the very best of my ability, to be the best mother I can be for him...

The beginning of my life was definitely the beginning of my mental health problems. I never felt right at school, in groups, always on the outside, but nobody would ever have known. I couldn't tell anyone and didn't trust anyone. If I tried to talk about it a bit with people, I was so dismissed that in the end I stopped. I find it so hard to trust anyone and expect everyone to leave me; nobody sticks around for me, especially if I am really me. It is a painful place to live. I'm in recovery from a multitude of addictions, which masked the mental illness and, as many people now acknowledge, addiction is also a mental illness... I have been diagnosed with chronic PTSD (Post Traumatic Stress Disorder), which relates to childhood trauma and I'm in therapy. I have been for eighteen years. I have had many therapists; a lot of them have not been right for me and that has caused me even more damage.

I look back and see so many turning points where things could have been easier for me. To have had parents who connected with me and understood the importance of being with their baby at the beginning, not working so hard all the time. Putting the baby first after they had me and getting to really know me and my needs and wondering why I was so aggressive at such a young age, instead of punishing me all the time and telling me how jealous I am of my brother. To have someone help me with understanding emotional things at a young age, and supporting me over a long time, would have really helped me; it was all piecemeal. My father not allowing my stepmother to be so unkind and actually doing something about that would have been massive. Then, as I grew and people saw there was a problem: instead of just seeing it, actually being there for me and talking and helping me.

I always felt like the life and soul of the party, which I was, but so lonely inside and now people tell me they had absolutely no idea, or they knew something was really wrong and didn't say anything. I had absolutely no idea what feelings were and if people did offer a bit of help, if I got too emotional they would just drop me; it was horrendous. I needed someone who knew the extent of my problems and who would listen and hold me, I needed a loving mummy who loved me unconditionally and who knew me; I still do.

Men thought it was Christmas around me; I was beautiful with such low self-esteem and thought that if a man wanted sex I had to give it to him. It was mayhem. I just gave myself away, it was what I thought I had to do.

I had stigma around me for many things: being wild, being unruly, being disruptive, being poor, being a single mum, being on welfare, being homeless, being crazy, being unstable and on it goes... all of which stem from feeling so desperate and feeling so unloved and unwanted and the extent of the trauma I suffered.

As I have got older it has got worse because my life has very slowly unravelled. I find that people are generally happy to be around me when I am happy and have something they want or reflect a certain status, but once I lost everything, I lost my so-called life. That was also one of the worst things, friends not understanding, not being able to cope with my brain unravelling in front of their eyes and my paranoia getting so bad.

I remember very clearly, a friend of mine and I had lunch in London, it was lovely and we had a good time. On the train home, my head was telling me (it's always my mother or stepmother's voice) how awful and fake I was and how, if she really knew me, she would hate me like everyone else hates me because I am such a bad and nasty person and all I was telling her was total lies. I believed them and rang my friend; she said she has no idea what I'm talking about, and that we had a great time. I believed them so much that when this happened again, she said she could not cope with it anymore, I lost a friend.

This happened a lot, especially when I started therapy in 1996. The voices in my head got louder and louder, it was a living hell. They are still there, even today, and I can't shut them up with booze anymore, so I have to ride them out. Sometimes it's so bad I'm literally holding on to the mattress for ages until they pass.

Other friends have been unable to stay around because they find me too deep or too challenging when I can't stand their behaviour and am honest about it. I have realised a lot of people really do not discuss their feelings, they just go along with it all, just like I used to, and I find it almost impossible to be around it anymore.

One of my friends said, "No way Penny, not you", when I told her I had clinical depression years ago. She said, "Come on, pull yourself up, I can't believe it, you have so much going for you, get a job, do something..." All the stuff that only made me feel even worse, because I was crippled with depression.

My mother told me to get off my lazy fat arse and get an f'ing job. I was utterly devastated, especially when she helped my brother so much later on. I was a single mum, I had just finished my film making degree and was unable to pursue my career, which was in itself devastating, especially as I had won awards for Fuji and had been to BAFTA to receive it. I had no family help or support and I saw my life slip through my fingers.

I went to the doctor's. She gave me an internal examination and asked me if I had been abused in my life. When I asked her what she was talking about, she said, "You tell me, emotionally, sexually or physically," and I said, "Try all three."

I was left with no therapist to help me for over six months. The only support I had was a CPN (Community Psychiatric Nurse) who came to visit me every week to ensure I was not dead and a social worker whom I was too scared to talk to because I was a single mum and terrified if I did tell her how bad it was, instead of helping me work through it, they would take my son away.

My friends still try to fix it today instead of listening to me and I have to say, it's one of the saddest things, being unseen by friends who you thought were your friends. It is a very lonely feeling.

I write a blog and am quite open about my life, but I do know that people go one of two ways: they either walk away, or a few walk closer. I'm learning very slowly to be more focused on the ones who walk towards me. My family have nothing to do with me; they all call me a drama queen and attention seeker.

I think the stigma is more subtle than a lot of people would understand or want to admit. I find a lot of people think they need to patronise me, talk down to me. A lot of stigma actually comes from the health professionals who have no real idea how to help and think they know what is best for me - they don't and they don't listen enough and ask the right questions because they are so convinced they know what to do and how to help. They often jump in, telling me what to think instead of just being able to listen; I find that one of the most horrendous forms of stigma. We are all different and the professionals have a huge amount to learn from us, it needs to be client led, not therapist imposed.

I realise I have not mentioned my current situation and the effects of the long term trauma on my mental health. As I got further into therapy, I became very unwell. One of the reasons for this was because I was in psychoanalysis and I have limited cognition for processing information; most people find processing concepts, when they are emotional, very hard. So for a start, I think psychoanalysis is not the right therapy for me.

I had several other therapists and, through the

journey, I realise that the relationship between the client and therapist is so vital for healing. I have also been restricted by funds and the offer of the NHS is very limited, CBT (Cognitive Behaviour Therapy) for twelve sessions would not touch the sides and did not touch the sides for me.

Building a long term, trusting relationship where healing and fear can be expressed in equal measures and to feel safe and understood with someone talking a language, on a level you understand, that for me is where the healing is. I still struggle with the therapy because of the damage done to me over a long time of misunderstanding; bringing the trauma up and then not being able to support me has done me untold damage.

Sometimes I wonder if I will ever get better but, for today, I have to believe that I am getting better. Learning to be there for myself and finding the right support for me is essential for my healing.

Short term therapy only makes people worse, in my opinion, because by the time they are beginning to connect with their feelings, they are told, "Time up." There is a huge divide within the therapy community: those who can afford it are open to incredible support, not always right, but they can afford the choice. If you are waiting for the NHS, or some other support, where there are long lists and short amount of support available, it can be very distressing. The right help at the right time would be the greatest solution for recovery.

Maisie's Story

STIGMA STILL STAYS

I watched the telly the other night and it was all about having something mentally wrong with you and how nobody wants to talk about it, especially family and friends. I thought to myself, I am fifty years old now and it was supposed to be better and more understood... Rubbish! It is exactly the same attitude now as it was thirty years ago, only they dress it up with different words, different therapies and different treatment.

The stigma still stays.

In my day, you didn't talk about wanting to smother your kid just to shut up the never ending crying and Jesus, you sure as hell never told *anybody* that you actually got up one night and tried to do it. However, I didn't know I was suffering from severe post natal depression, or baby blues, as we called it then. I was just terrified that I was evil, wicked and at the very least, abnormal.

If you were abnormal, then they took your kids away from you and you could be sectioned at the nearest mental hospital and stay there forever. I had heard the stories so I knew it happened. When I couldn't stop my baby son from crying, all day and all night, I told the antenatal clinic and the nurse there said I would just have to be patient and he would settle down. If he wasn't hungry or wet then just lie him down and ignore him, he would soon learn to stop crying. I wanted to tell her about putting the pillow over his face but I knew it could mean losing him and I did love him. But I was so tired from not having any sleep and my husband was useless, never waking up through it all and telling me that I was probably doing something wrong…

I didn't tell, or want anyone to know that I wasn't doing the washing; I was piling it in the bins, not even rinsing out the dirty nappies and when I had run out of all the baby clothes, I would go out and buy new ones. I just couldn't face that overflowing bin or the slow building up of plastic bags, hidden in cupboards or under the stairs. I remember one day, I was so ashamed of what I was doing that I attempted to empty one bag and the nappies fell out, with maggots falling everywhere. I had to be sick and after that, I burned them in the garden.

One day I got the six-monthly visit from the health visitor and, when she asked if I had any problems, I somehow plucked up the courage to tell her about how I couldn't cope and how I shut him in another room so I couldn't hear him. She suggested I change over his milk powder and then I blurted out what I had tried to do to him. She looked quite horrified for a moment and then said, "Well dear, the important thing is that you didn't do it, you stopped yourself and you are an intelligent young lady and realise that it would have been a criminal act and, of course, we would have had to take your baby away from you; which I am sure you don't want to happen. So I will send in another health visitor next week just to check up how you are doing."

And that was it. I couldn't believe that she was, in effect, doing nothing and leaving my baby to a possible murderess, just because I had told her and that I had stopped myself from harming him. The thing was, I really did want her to take him away from me because I just didn't want to cope anymore.

I then made the mistake of telling my friend what I had done. She was horrified and disgusted with me and wasted no time in telling me so. I never saw her again after that and I felt that I was a really bad person if she didn't want to know or try to understand what was happening to me. I was so ashamed and promised myself I would never, ever, tell anyone again. It was my secret and I would hide it from everyone. I succeeded too.

I would shut my son in his bedroom and leave him for at least an hour crying and then I would pick him up and walk around the house, leaning him over my shoulder and rubbing his back and if the weather was nice, I would go into the garden, still holding him. He never stopped crying though and it continued for nearly a year. I was worn out, angry. I felt useless and my moods swung from self hatred to dreadful guilt and down into sheer hopelessness. I never went out and would never let people into my home. I then began to get up later and later, doing nothing at all until half an hour before my husband came home. Then I would rush round to get dinner on and try to do the washing up. By the time he came in, everything seemed normal and he didn't bother about his son crying upstairs in his bedroom, or ever ask why.

I really don't remember how I carried on for the next year, I only know it wasn't me living in that house, doing those things, it was someone else pretending to be me and I could never let anyone else know about it. I think I had two health visits in all that time but maybe because I took my son to the monthly clinic, after washing him and putting new clothes on him each time and smiling and saying all was well, they didn't feel I was a risk factor.

I remember one day I realised that my son hadn't cried for a whole morning. I picked him up out of his cot and he was looking at me, instead of his face being screwed up and crying. I took him downstairs and put him on the settee and then I started to talk to him and all of a sudden he smiled. It was so beautiful and I held him to me and couldn't stop crying. After all my shouting and screaming at him, all my closing him out, my baby could still smile at me and I felt that he at least had forgiven me.

From that day on, something changed forever and slowly I began to find the energy to begin to put my home in order, clean up the filth, clean up myself too. Whatever it was that was wrong with my son, (or indeed, was it what was wrong with me all along?) I will never know, but slowly I got better and I learned to love my child again.

I have, however, never learned to forgive myself and I have never got over the shame. I also know that were I to share this with anyone else, even today, there would probably be horror and disgust on their part and I know that they would never look at me in quite the same way again.

Mental illness has a stigma and will always have a stigma. I don't believe it will ever change. Only when it affects people personally will they begin to understand a little better maybe, but they will still continue to hide it from others.

And so it goes on.

Breaking The Silence

Daniel's Story

On reflection I just wonder. I wonder whether I have experienced the isolation, the sense of perceived desertion, almost betrayal, that can often accompany the stigmatisation of mental health.

I had been Headteacher of the school for twelve years. No ordinary school, one which was an integral part of an adolescent mental health inpatient unit. The school had gone from strength to strength, receiving recognition for the outstanding quality of learning it provided young people who were experiencing crises in their lives. Over the years I had built around me a wonderful team of experienced and thoroughly professional staff who were strongly united in working towards a common goal: offering compassionate support to our students, assisting in helping them to reconstruct their lives and enabling them to believe that there was hope for their futures. It was an immense privilege to work in such a unique setting away from the "factory" type learning environment of most secondary schools, where the focus is upon results and not having the time to develop the unique qualities and skills of each and every student.

The school was part of a wonderful team of highly talented, multi-disciplinary professionals, all operating in a supportive environment and working towards enabling the recovery of each young person in our care.

My staff, without exception, were highly talented and exceptionally skilled practitioners who provided exemplary support for our students. Being a small team and working so closely together, it felt like we were almost a "family". I felt I was not only amongst colleagues but individuals who over the years had become friends. That was, until my health began to change. Increasingly exhausted by ridiculously long hours and striving to ever improve the work of my school, the "batteries" began to run low. Eventually my reserves were exhausted and I had no choice but to take time off work. I knew at the time that my career of thirty-six years in teaching was, sadly, coming to an end.

On the one hand I wanted to isolate myself from everyone from school but at the same time I craved for my colleagues to contact me, to show their concern and perhaps offer their support. Not all that dissimilar from the type of support we offered our students on a daily basis. Sadly, I received no such contact as not one of my colleagues tried to contact me, to reach out in my time of need.

Now, it may be that I had got things very wrong. Perhaps they did not feel the friendship I thought we had developed. But I just wonder. I wonder whether, despite the fact we were all working so skilfully within the world of young peoples' mental health, we were unable to transfer and employ those skills to the adult world. That a member of staff, particularly the Headteacher should experience even a relatively mild episode of mental health problems was something that even skilled practitioners working in the world of mental health were just unable to respond to, unable to handle in an empathetic manner.

So, I just wonder, following my experience, what it is like for others who suffer from mental health issues. If highly trained and experienced individuals do not have the understanding of how to respond to a colleague or friend, what must it be like for those who find themselves dependent, in a time of crisis, solely upon the help of strangers to support them in their hour of need?

Emma's Story

I am a thirty-five-year-old current service user. I was first introduced to the mental health services at the age of thirteen and I have been in and out of services since.

I volunteer with the Trust and have been involved with many opportunities, but the one I have the most passion for is sharing my own story, in the hope that I can change people's views and show them the importance of how we should all be working with recovery as our main focus.

I also write an award-winning blog and own a large support group, for mothers with a mental illness, on Facebook.

Oh and I also have six children.

I have since bought some TVs and when people comment on how many children I have with, "Are you crazy", I smile and nod.

Let me share with you my own story as a service user and why I believe recovery needs to be the main focus when treating us.

Almost five years ago I found myself standing on a bridge; I was also holding onto the hand of my two-year-old daughter.

I DON'T BELIEVE I WANTED TO DIE; I JUST DIDN'T WANT TO HURT ANYMORE

I couldn't do it, no matter how low I felt I couldn't kill my child, she saved me that day.

I will never forget the look on my husband's face when I returned home and told him what I had almost done; it still haunts me to this day and I still struggle to bond with my daughter whom I almost killed.

I became angry; why the hell was there no help out there?

I had asked for help, but there was nobody willing to listen.

And so I visited the GP again, I was given more antidepressants and made to feel this was all very normal. I had postnatal depression he told me, medication would help me.

I didn't have much hope, I had been on antidepressants for most of my life.

I didn't tell him about what had happened on the bridge or about the voices I heard, mostly telling me to hurt my children. I didn't tell him about the people and animals I saw or about the need to harm myself; he didn't give me chance to.

Part of me feared what they would do to me if I was honest, would they take my children away or would they section me?

To be honest, looking back that would have been the safest option for me and those around me.

Despite the fear, I was at rock bottom and I was ready to be honest but nobody wanted to listen to me, or give me chance to speak.

HE JUST PLACED YET ANOTHER PRESCRIPTION IN MY HAND

I didn't return to the GP for a long time after that; what was the point?

Anyway, I continued on a roller coaster ride and went onto have my fifth baby. The mania allowed me to stay afloat: three days after giving birth, I started my fourth business.

Voices and visions began hounding my waking hours and my nightmares became my reality. They criticised, threatened and wanted me to harm my children.

I was afraid, alone and failed by a system that was meant to help me.

Banging my head off the wall, watching as the blood ran from my nose, I felt relief. The physical pain I inflicted upon myself stopped the mental pain, if only for a few minutes.

Finding out I was pregnant again wasn't a shock, I was hardly acting responsibly at this time. This would be my third baby in three years.

I started to believe that I was being followed wherever I went; there was no rest from the torture, even in the bath I would feel that hand coming towards me, pushing me under the water, thrashing about and then gasping for air.

WAS I TRYING TO DROWN MYSELF OR HAD SOMEONE HELD ME UNDER?

My eldest daughter, who would have been twelve at the time, had witnessed this a few times and to this day she still comes and sits in the bathroom when I go for a bath; she suffered horrific nightmares after these events and, though she knows I was poorly at the time, she still worries.

I was angry at the world, at the system, at myself and I am not proud to admit that I became aggressive to my husband.

While most mothers pray that the Lord keeps their children safe at night, I was praying that He would take me and end my pain.

My husband was at breaking point; he spoke with my health visitor.

Thanks to her I agreed to see a different GP, she promised to come with me; she did. I was referred to the mental health team, finally.

She went above and beyond her job title; if guardian angels exist then she is mine.

I was assessed by the Crisis Team and passed onto someone else, who told me he couldn't help me as I needed secondary services.

AND SO I WAITED FOR ANOTHER APPOINTMENT

I saw a peri-natal psychiatrist a number of times during my pregnancy, she believed I had Cyclothymia; I didn't hear the L in the word and thought she said I had pyscho themia and I was horrified that I was indeed a Pyscho after all.

I refused to take the Lithium and preferred to be drug free during the pregnancy.

But despite being honest about the voices and the visions when I was admitted to hospital with exhaustion, I was placed on a maternity ward with five other women.

The voices told me to hurt the other women and their babies.

When I asked a midwife for a knife so I could cut out my own baby, she went to fetch someone. After a little chat he deemed me safe and suggested something to help me sleep. I took his word for it, I mean, you trust the health professionals don't you?

My baby was born and I was discharged. My father and stepmother moved in with us for three months. I wasn't able to look after myself, let alone six children.

I was assigned my first CPN. I would arrive for appointments and sit in reception for what felt like a lifetime before the receptionist would come and tell me that she was off sick that day.

I had a case open with Social Services at this time over access arrangements for my three eldest children to see their father.

CaffCass had reported him to be a danger if left unsupervised with them, yet the social worker believed my mental health was clouding my judgement of him and questioned whether I was meeting the emotional needs of my children.

I had spent eleven years being beaten, raped and mentally tortured by this man. The Social worker took none of the police and medical reports into account.

My CPN knew about the abusive history and I had begged her to come with me. She never turned up for the final meeting and I sat there alone, humiliated and unable to speak out for myself. He won unsupervised access.

On the third weekend of unsupervised contact taking place the police returned my children; they were too traumatised to even speak. They have not seen their father in over a year now.

That social worker had used my mental illness against me and put my children in danger and, yes, I was angry at my CPN; but I never had chance to tell her because at my next appointment a new CPN was there.

She liked cats – that's all I can really tell you about our six month professional relationship.

I didn't have the strength to go through it all again to get nowhere. I had lost my faith in the system. I pretended everything was fine. She discharged me.

I returned to the mental health team some months later. This time I was informed I would see the new CPN who had joined the local team. I disliked him before I even met him; he was just going to let me down, like all the others had.

I arrived to that appointment and, you guessed it, this new CPN wasn't able to see me, he had been called away due to an emergency.

I remember a "small drama" followed, resulting in me screaming and shouting at the poor receptionist, telling her how useless the mental health system was. She nodded and smiled at me, the first person to smile at me for a long time.

Most people feared me, my moods and behaviour were unpredictable. I had lost my career, some family members had turned their backs on me because I embarrassed them and my best friend at the time didn't want her children around me. I had drained the bank account and had to be supervised at all times.

But that receptionist didn't fear me, she saw a vulnerable women screaming out for help and she found someone who would see me. There was a psychiatrist available and she asked him to see me immediately and he agreed.

I don't really remember what happened, I was pretty much hysterical but he made a phone call to the psychiatrist who had previously prescribed me medication; I wasn't to take that again. I would become his patient from then on in and I'm so glad

I met him that day.

I was fast tracked an appointment with this new CPN and he did turn up and has done ever since. It took a long time for me to trust him, but he was patient and I learned to respect him.

Not only has he given me back my faith in the mental health system, he saved my life.

He didn't judge me; he actually listened and advised, but allowed me to voice my own opinion.

I told him about the voices and visions, how I self-harmed and self-starved myself and how I self-medicated with Tramadol.

He didn't look at me in disgust as many friends had; he explained that it was all part of my illness.

I wasn't a Psycho after all, I had bipolar.

Strangely, as it turned out I had many female relatives diagnosed with manic depression. It's a huge taboo in my family and now I know why they turned their backs on me, they were afraid.

I told my CPN about my fear of medications and he talked through everything with me. I no longer felt a freak; I actually started to believe that I could live with this condition after all, with the correct support in place.

AND THIS IS WHERE MY RECOVERY BEGAN

He told me that recovery was not only possible, it would happen for me but I had to do that part for myself.

But as my recovery began, the devastation I had caused was soul-destroying, I almost lost everything.

I had six children whom I had no idea how to interact with, I felt such a failure. I had no idea how to begin to explain how I had become a stranger to them. My husband had raised them alone for three years, with me in the background.

Have you any idea how it feels to have your children ask you why you don't love them anymore?

I had spent so long pushing them away, locking myself away for weeks at a time.

I needed to make them not need me so I was able to take my own life without feeling guilty. If they didn't love me then my death wouldn't hurt them and they wouldn't miss me.

The truth is I resented them, they prevented my suicide. I blamed them for the pain I felt, I wanted that pain to end but I couldn't end it because of them.

My CPN involved a service who were amazing and gave us family therapy and I am pleased to say my relationship with my children is stronger than ever.

My husband and I are still together, he has his own counsellor now too. He had to give up his career to become my full-time carer, he's my best friend who has stood beside me all of the way, he never gave up on me when others did.

You see, it's all good and well treating the diagnosis but so much more happens in a service user's life.

My friendships were destroyed, career over, my marriage was torn to shreds, finances crumbled and I no longer had any sense of my own identity.

I HAD TO PICK UP THE PIECES AND BEGIN TO REBUILD MY LIFE

And medication can only do so much.

Now I have been far from the model patient, I have pushed health professionals to their limits so many times. But my CPN earned my respect and trust and we have a great professional relationship.

When I told him I was joining the Trust to save the world, he just tutted, he's used to my grand gestures these days.

But he was surprised when I told him I had spent a

week working with my own psychiatrist on a project.

All the anger I felt towards the mental health system faded when my own psychiatrist personally apologised for the way the system had failed me. Although it was not his doing, he admitted there were many faults.

He also suggested I get more involved because he believed I would be a great asset to the Trust.

I began writing about my personal journey four years ago. I have met so many service users and carers who share their own experiences on the blog too.

I am sorry that my recovery took so long; so many health professionals failed me when I needed them most.

I LOST THREE YEARS OF LIFE

I have no idea what my youngest children's first words were, how old they were when they first crawled or walked, those are moments I will never get back.

I, of course, would prefer to live a life without a mental illness yet it's who and what I am and I have finally accepted that, I can now laugh at my "quirkiness traits".

And I have learned that I can stay bitter and angry or I can use my experience in a positive way to help others and that is what I am now doing.

I am living proof that we can recover and recovery should have been the focus for me at the very start.

I was made to feel that I was stuck this way, that nothing would ever change for me and I would be this way for life; no wonder I stood on that bridge.

It took years and numerous health professionals to find one who believed in me and saw me as a person and not just a diagnosis. He didn't believe that just medicating me was the answer; he taught me and gave me the tools I needed to live with my illness.

I do wish I had met him sooner, all staff should be this way, is it really just a job to them? Didn't they choose this career to help people recover and live a happy and fulfilled life?

While I agree medication plays a big part in recovery, it cannot be the only option.

Learning to accept your diagnosis can be traumatic and peer support should be introduced to the service, being given a key worker who can truly relate to you would be a lifesaving tool.

Sometimes all we need is an ear to listen and

shoulder to lean on.

Speaking to other service users and carers is what has personally helped me. Knowing I am not alone and have someone to talk to who really does understand, means I no longer have to go to that dark place again.

You can recover from mental illness and recovery means different things to different people.

For me it means I am no longer afraid to wake each morning. I now have hopes and dreams and I can plan for my future.

I have learned that recovery is something you have to achieve for yourself. It is not something that someone else does for you, but you do need support from health professionals along this journey.

And that's the thing with recovery, there is no destination, you don't suddenly become well again, it truly is a journey.

For me, I will always have bipolar and the voices and visions are still very present.

I have not self-harmed for over eighteen months now and I know that self-starving myself isn't the answer, I do have more control now.

I am still addicted to Tramadol and that's another battle I have to face, but I am no longer a victim, I am a survivor and I have a great support system in place now.

I know my journey will still come across bumps in the roads and I still have a few mountains to climb, I just hope to avoid the bridges along the way.

Recovery is a way of living a satisfying, hopeful and contributing life even with the limitations caused by illness.

DON'T WE DESERVE THAT?

I hope, by sharing my own experience, at least one of you will begin to look at recovery as being the most important aspect in our treatment.

To support recovery, professionals need to work in partnership with service users and carers, making joint decisions about what treatment is appropriate, rather than 'knowing what is best'.

We can recover; we just need someone to help us and someone to believe in us. This is our life we place in their hands.

Breaking The Silence

Maria's Story

At the age of sixteen I experienced my first manic episode. It was said to have been caused by a knock to the head when I was involved in a serious car accident in Belgium when I was ten. The doctors in Belgium, when they heard the news about my mental state, were not surprised and said that they were waiting for that to happen. They said, because of the injury to my frontal lobe, it was expected that at some period during my life I would experience some sort of episode. This only came to light because the case for the medical injury claim was still going through in Belgium.

The episode started just before I was due to take my GCSE's. It was believed that it was triggered by the stress of the exams, although I felt I experienced no stress at all really.

One night I was taken to hospital, as my mum didn't know what was wrong with me. My uncle was with us too. I was put in an ambulance and taken to a mental health unit. In the ambulance there was the sound of an alarm, it sounded exactly like the alarm at school. At the place the ambulance took me to, where we were waiting for me to be seen, there was this vending machine; I had a peanut butter KitKat and a packet of crisps. I had this delusion that I was in heaven, and my family were too. I was taken to this place called New Beginnings and had to stay there. I had my own room. That place had other young people there around my age. It was a terrible place. I felt like I was in prison being tortured and felt I had to escape. One night I made a run for it but all the main doors were locked so I couldn't go out anywhere. I ran past the nurses and the night staff. They got me and took me back to my room. They had this orange looking liquid and tried to force it down me. It ended up going all over my face as I refused to take it, I shut my lips so tight. I didn't know what it was for at that time, I didn't know what they were forcing me to take. As it was all on my face it burned, I felt this horrible burning sensation. I went and washed my face. In the room I was staying, there was a bathroom. The first time I used it, all I remember is this man and woman trying to shower me, I felt like I was drowning and was so afraid of the water.

There were a few incidents that happened where I was treated atrociously. There was this one incident I call 'the bean bag incident'. I saw that one of the carers was really bothering this girl and being quite horrible so I said to her "You're upsetting her, leave her alone she just wants to be left alone." That was it. They dragged me to a small box room with large bean bags in. On the other side of the door was a carer pushing the door closed. She had her back to it sitting down. I was shouting, "Let me out!" But I got nothing and carried on shouting "Let me out!" But still nothing. As they were refusing to do so, I tore all the bean bags and emptied out all their contents. Still nothing, though I was still in there and just wanted to escape and felt extremely claustrophobic. I managed to prise the door open, that woman was quite large. I put my fingers in the gap I had opened to try and force it open but she pushed back on the door squashing my fingers flat but I then managed to force the door open again and this time managed to get out. I ran as fast as I could go and jumped on the seats in the communal area. What happened after that I only remember vaguely. All I do remember is being so distressed, I just wanted to be free from that horrible place.

Two other memories I have, not sure which one happened first. One time I was in the "quiet room" and this guy was with me, I think he was a psychologist or something like that. He asked me to close my eyes, asking, "What colours do you see?" I said "Purple." This was a relaxation thing, I guess.

The other memory I have is of being extremely distressed. I was on the floor, pulling at this doctor's tie. I had such a tight grip and wouldn't let go, he went so red. They managed to finally get me to let go. I only remember bits and pieces of what I went through in that place.

I was sitting down in the communal area with the others. We were having a session. Suddenly, for no reason, this male nurse came over to me grabbed me by the wrist, got me up, twisting my arm, dragging me to this other room. I was put in there with two of the staff. I was trapped in there with them, not allowed to escape. After the bean bag incident my parents insisted on taking me home as they were not happy with the way I was being treated. They said to my dad that if he was to take me home they would call the police. He said that he didn't care if they called them, he was taking me home.

I was then a day patient. My mum would take me there in the morning and come to collect me later.

There were times at that place where I wanted to call my mum but they wouldn't let me. One time I really wanted to call my mum. This woman in the office there refused. I was so anxious I needed to call my mum, but still she refused. I went on and on pleading with her for me to make that call. Eventually she let me. I was so relieved to hear my mum's voice.

I don't know why I was treated that way. Was I treated that way because of my mental state? Did they not know how to deal with me? I wasn't even allowed out with the staff when the others were. Why I was treated that way I do not know, all I know is that it has scarred me forever.

I got my first job working as a carer in a social educational place for people with autism and learning disabilities. I volunteered for a few weeks and then was given the job. I loved working there, the only time I felt like I belonged. I've always felt different, like an outcast. Ever since I can remember I knew I was different from all the other kids. My mum believed that I had ADHD as I was so disruptive and extremely hyper. I would tear up classmates' work, hit the teachers and have my shoes confiscated from me. My mum took me from doctor to doctor but all they could say was that there was nothing wrong with me and it was all in her head. Anyway, at this place, I felt so comfortable and I felt that I finally fitted in somewhere and could relate to others.

Unfortunately, a week after I got the job the boss's best friend, who was the receptionist, took a dislike to me and I was told that I no longer had the job. Well, that's the reason I believe to be true because I can't think of any other one. I tried to explain to the boss that the job meant everything to me, and me being too honest as always I told her about my mental health. She carried on saying that she had to let me go. She then used what I said to her about my mental health against me and turned that into the reason why she let me go. She said to me, "If a client were to have an epileptic fit you wouldn't know what to do," meaning that I wouldn't know how to communicate to the other staff. I knew that what she was saying to me, she was only saying it and not meaning it. She just wanted me gone and used my mental health as an excuse. She said that I could come back in six months if I kept my mouth shut and not tell the other carers why I lost my job. Which I stupidly believed.

The other staff there were shocked to find out that I had lost my job. A senior staff member said to me how well I was doing. I had to lie to them and say that the job was getting to me. Which is the lie she wanted me to say. I hate lying, I am a truthful person. It's a gift and a curse. I only said that to them because of what she said to me about coming back. In her words, "If you tell them, the gates will be closed," meaning I wouldn't be able to return, "but if you don't tell them the gates will be open." Losing the job that I loved felt like I had my heart ripped out, I was so angry and upset.

A couple of days later, my mum saw an ad in the newspaper about needing support workers in a care home for young adults with autism between the ages of sixteen and twenty-five. As nervous as I was, I rang up straight away. When I was interviewed I was honest and told them about the knock to my head (frontal lobe) and said how I find it difficult processing information and other ways it affects me. I walked away thinking, too honest again as usual. I got a call a couple of days after from the manager saying that they can offer me part time. I thought to myself, ah, what I told them affected me getting the full time job. I said yes, sure, thank you.

My first day was terrible; brought back memories from New Beginnings. I was shadowing two female staff supporting 'Sarah'. I was disgusted at the way they were treating her. Shadowing, all I could do was watch as I felt so intimidated by them, they were just horrible. Sarah dropped something she was holding onto the floor. They said to her in a nasty tone, "Pick that up, Sarah. Pick that up, now. Pick it up!" When she didn't pick it up, they got her and forced her head down to the floor at what she had dropped, her face almost touching it. I was horrified, and felt scared, not just for me but for Sarah. It took me straight back to how I was treated. My mind blocked out the trauma of seeing that, maybe did so as a way of coping. Being there was a constant reminder of New Beginnings. I took care of 'Alfie' too, who was also mistreated, which leads me to my second episode.

All the service users had to be watched by staff constantly. Alfie had chronic tonic epilepsy. Out of the service users he was neglected the most. He would be left alone in his flat. While he would be in his room the staff would sit in his living room and constantly watch TV. On one occasion, Alfie had a fit and the staff member who was meant to be looking after him was not there to support him as he fell. Because of that Alfie took knocks to the head.

Alfie would be left to tear up a large amount of his photos his family had given him. I reported that to Management but it didn't stop straight away. One incident that happened was the cause of my recurring episode. I was in the park with Sam who was a fellow staff member and James, a service user. Suddenly I heard Alfie and saw him running away from the staff members who were with him. Alfie was running about and the staff with him were trying to get him to stop. One of them, Gloria, struck at him a few times with her umbrella. I looked at Sam with disbelief. I was so shocked to see what had just happened, my mind immediately blocked it out.

I don't remember why, but a week later Gloria got confrontational with me. She came really close to me, intimidating me. I honestly thought she was going to hit me. Suddenly a flashback came to me of her hitting Alfie. I informed staff of what she had done to Alfie and straight away she lost her job. I still was concerned with the way Alfie was being treated, I felt that he was being neglected. Which he was, in my eyes. The Deputy Manager advised me to whistle blow. Well, she asked me to. She said she would do it but it wouldn't look good coming from her. I said that I'll do it when I get home, so I did. My second episode shortly followed. I thought that they were going to use my mental health against me and say that I had made it up or imagined it. But it was taken seriously, and an investigation was carried out.

Six months had passed so I called the boss from my previous job. She had said I could come back if I hadn't said anything to anyone. I thought she'd take me back. I called, she answered. I asked about me going back and she said no, this job isn't for you. I knew straight away she was saying that because of what I had told her about my mental health. As soon as I put the phone down I cried. My mum phoned her back and asked her what had just happened and wanted to find out why I had broken into tears. She said exactly what she had said to me, but she wouldn't give a true explanation as to why.

In my head I feel that people who know about my mental health treat me differently. I feel that they treat me as if I'm fragile and have to be careful not to break me. I feel that they talk to me differently from how they would talk to someone else. I feel this a lot with my family. Maybe it is in my head, or maybe it's not. I'll never truly know.

Mental health problems are invisible, people still don't truly understand and I feel that they never will. I've always said that people only truly understand if they've been through it themselves.

I feel that medical professionals still don't fully understand mental illness and its effects on people who suffer it. I've seen my fair share of doctors, consultants and therapists and it's very rare to find those who do have an understanding of their patients. I've seen a few therapists through my hard times when struggling mentally. I was lucky to have had one therapist, the most recent one, who had been fantastic in that he would show an understanding of what I had discussed with him. My current consultant, however, whom I started seeing after I was passed over from the home treatment team following my second episode, has no understanding whatsoever about me and the problems I am experiencing and have experienced. During my first episode I wanted a diagnosis of what I was going through, I wanted to know what was 'wrong' with me. I saw a consultant at the Priory and was diagnosed with Bipolar Disorder. I was happy that I had finally put a name to what I was going through. I feel that the consultant I am seeing now doesn't actually know how to handle me. She has no understanding at all about what to do with me. She doesn't understand me. She keeps on saying that I don't have Bipolar, I have Borderline Personality Disorder. When she says that to me I feel so annoyed, how can she just say that when it is clear that she just doesn't understand? I feel certain that I have Bipolar Disorder, not just because my dad has it, too. It is important to me that I do have a label to what I have, even though what I have does not define who I am. It just defines how I may act.

Colin's Story

Leaving school should have been a relief. I was a mediocre student in an all-boys' grammar school, was hopeless at cricket and rugby (the school's other routes to success), and was good only at being the school clown. Even in the Sixth Form I had no motivation. I hated the pointlessness of school rules, did the minimum amount of homework I could get away with and was bored silly with History lessons. And as for the Jane Austen book I was expected to read and comment on for A level English, I managed to read half a page before giving up on it, bored witless.

So my departure from that exalted place of learning must have been as blessed a relief for the schoolmasters there as it ought to have been for me.

But at the age of eighteen, when many of my schoolmates were embarking on university or college courses and taking the first steps towards an eventual career, I had no idea what to do with my life. My exam results had been predictably poor and gave me few options of any value.

To add to all this were two other factors: having attended an all-boys' school I had no skills at all with women; and having been brought up in a mainstream Jewish family, I felt I didn't fit well into the world around me. I was the proverbial fish out of water.

I was suffering from severe depression and it began to distress my mother. My dad, probably worrying more about her than about me, suggested I go and see our family doctor. After having a chat with me and prescribing some pills whose name I've forgotten, he arranged for me to see a psychiatrist.

The psychiatrist who interviewed me was not only a member of our local Jewish community – he was also a friend of my parents. I can't recall much of what I told him but I do remember him rolling his eyes at one point and saying dismissively, "Well, we all feel like that..."

He must have taken me more seriously than that sounds, though, because the outcome of the meeting was a prolonged stay of about three months in a mental hospital out in the country. It wasn't a bad place to be in some respects. I was well treated in personal terms. However, I was in a ward where the treatment meant being put into a daily coma by means of insulin injections. We were brought round after a few hours with a sugar solution piped up our noses. To this day, years later, I have no idea of what this was supposed to achieve.

Whatever it was meant to do, it evidently failed in

my case because I was then given a couple of sessions of ECT (electro-convulsive therapy). All I recall of these were the headaches: the headache after ECT was the granddaddy of *all* headaches. For a while after coming round from the treatment I didn't even know my own name, let alone where I was. The other effect was that much of my memory remained, and still remains, lost in mist. Occasionally the mist clears a little and a few wisps of memory drift by. Some parts of my earlier life still stand like mountain peaks above a shroud of cloud but for the most part my childhood exists in my head only in fragments.

Eventually I left the hospital and started looking around for a job or, preferably, a career. For no reason I can recall, I decided on becoming a trainee store manager and filled in application forms to three major department stores.

The father of a friend warned me, "Don't tell them anything about your mental health treatment. It will go against you." That sounded a bit over the top to my ears. Why would anyone think any less of you for having treatment for any health problems, mental or physical?

None of the application forms had asked about my health but one did ask my religion. I answered truthfully, Jewish. I heard no more from them. It was much later on in life that I discovered they had an anti-Semitic policy.

The second form got me an interview at the company's head office in London. All seemed to be going well until I was asked what I'd done since leaving school. Choosing to forget the warning I'd been given by my friend's dad, I mentioned my hospitalisation. And that was the end of that opportunity.

I was called for interview by the third company. This time I resolved to keep quiet about anything to do with mental health. Greatly to my relief, I was given the job of trainee manager at a large department store in the Midlands.

Four months into the job, which I was quite enjoying, I let slip to a colleague that I'd been in hospital with depression. News travels fast in enclosed institutions and, within a couple of hours, I was in the manager's office being told that they were giving me a fortnight's salary in lieu of notice. All my protestations fell on deaf ears. I was escorted off the premises through the back entrance, presumably in case I contaminated anyone else. A promising career was ended before it had even begun properly.

For a few months I did very little, apart from meet friends in coffee bars. Eventually, my dad took matters into his own hands and pulled a few strings (he had a lot of friends and acquaintances).

"Any job's better than none," he told me. "I've arranged for you to have an interview at the local education offices."

The interview was with the local Director of Education himself. I said nothing about my mental health history and was given a job as what was known as a student teacher. What it actually meant was that I was an unqualified teacher who could take classes for a short stretch at a time, the idea being apparently to give such staff a taste of what teaching was like, in the hope they would want to take it further and gain teaching qualifications.

To my own surprise, I enjoyed the whole experience. I found the staff supportive and friendly and was accepted by the children, with whom I gained a generally good working relationship, despite the occasional discipline problems.

I applied to a teacher training college and was accepted, *subject to medical checks...*

I made an urgent appointment to see my GP and asked him to support my application by not divulging anything about my mental health problems.

"I'm sorry," he said. "What you're asking goes against medical ethics. But I won't lay it on too thick and I'll explain that you are now fully recovered."

Relieved, I put the whole thing to the back of my mind and continued with my life as normal – until a letter arrived from the College of Education informing me that their offer of a place was being withdrawn, owing to...

You guessed it!

I was heartbroken. For the first time in my life I actually had a burning ambition; and the opportunity I needed to make it a reality had been dangled before me, then snatched away.

It wasn't fair! *Life* wasn't fair! If there *was* a God, He was having a great laugh at my expense.

My dad, however, was not a person to accept life's knocks without putting up a fight and went to our Member of Parliament, who must have pulled a few of his own strings; this led to me being assessed by a psychiatrist. The result of his assessment was a clean bill of health. When I submitted the psychiatrist's report to the College, it did the trick – I was enrolled onto their teacher-training course for the following year. It was, admittedly, a year later than originally planned but it came as a huge relief.

From then on, I have kept my medical history to myself – after all, who wants their child being taught by a *nutter*? It's a sad reflection on the perceptions of those who have never suffered from mental health problems (or rather, those who have never had one *labelled* as such) that they regard anyone who has had such difficulties as being forever marked out as *weird, mad, fruitcakes...*

The truth is that if you could see inside the head of anyone else, you would be looking at an alien landscape. To each one of us, *all* the rest therefore would appear "weird". And yet somehow the human race continues to function.

I have been a successful qualified teacher for several years and have risen to the position of deputy head of a large primary school. I am well respected by my colleagues, as well as by parents and children, and do not see myself as anything but normal. But if I were ever to tell anyone that I once spent several months in a mental health unit..!

I sometimes wonder how many others out there are harbouring similar dark secrets. I've seen in my own life how quickly and easily the cold fingers of stigma can grab you by the throat and shake you. Sadly, I think if anything is to change, it will do so only very slowly.

But books like this one will help the process...

Amy Jean's Story

This isn't going to be easy for me to write…

There is always a reason for everything that happens to us. These reasons can have a huge impact on our mental and physical health. It did for me.

Sudden and drastic changes at the tender age of only seven and later, in my youth, caused severe changes in my personality. My development was affected also and therefore made it difficult for me to cope with life well.

As a result of the traumatic events, which were relentless, I ended up having a huge mental breakdown at around the age of twenty. Whilst in the psychiatric clinic, I suffered more sexual abuse at the hands of a male nurse. But nobody was listening to me. The staff put it down to my mental illness - one of my first serious experiences of STIGMA!

They just kept drugging me up to the eyeballs to keep me quiet. I was like a zombie! The abuse went on right up until I was discharged. It was awful! Tragic!

My bad experiences in care only added to the pain that I carried right through my life up until this present day. Now, I am helping in "Breaking the Silence". The time has come, at last, to break free and help others in the process.

Here is my story…

It wasn't an easy time for my mother when she got pregnant with me. She told me that she had been thinking of leaving Dad, so the news of my being was not at all welcomed. In fact, Mum told me, Dad was at his worst. He was more violent towards her; more than any other time.

Dad also was not pleased about her pregnancy. This only annoyed him more. So he drank to soothe himself. Ironically, the alcohol made him more stressed and angry!

What was about to happen to my mother, in the seven years to come, was to have devastating consequences for both Mum and for me also. Mum herself always encouraged me to write about my experience, just as I remember it.

During the last seven years of Mum and Dad living together, I witnessed some horrific scenes of extreme violence. This started right from me being in my mother's womb.

Mother told me of a time when she opened the car door on her side, so she could throw herself out to escape more punches from Dad. She was five months pregnant with me. Despite Dad being aware of Mum being with child, he continued to hit her hard repeatedly whilst still driving. Mum and I were both lucky to be alive!

Another occasion when Mum was still pregnant with me, Dad had chased her upstairs into my two older sisters' bedroom. Mum tried to hide under the bed to protect herself from his violence. Dad, being a very strong man, lifted the bed up, so Mum told me, and my sisters rolled out of it. Dad then grabbed my mother and as he beat her he had no regard for her well being, or my sisters. Sadly too, he didn't care for the safety of his unborn daughter, who was so small, so precious in my mother's womb. Me!!

The stress of Dad's violent behaviour made Mum very depressed. She told me that she tried to abort me, by getting into a very hot bath, as hot as she could bear. Then she drank a lot of alcohol at the same time. She had hoped that this would have caused her to miscarry me. Then she could leave Dad.

God had other plans, as here I am telling my story.

My memories of any good times do exist. There

were some happy holidays by the seaside. Also some nice moments shared with both Mum and Dad and my sisters. But they are vague. However, the bad experiences remain quite clear, enough to haunt me, sometimes on a daily basis. This makes my life very difficult to live at times.

Two other awful experiences I do remember, when Dad was violent to my mother, were when I was woken up to my mother screaming. She locked herself in the bathroom to hide from Dad. But he was so angry that he broke the door down and beat her. I, at that stage, had wandered onto the landing holding my teddy Rupert. I witnessed awful violence through tearful eyes. I wanted to protect Mummy but I was too small and afraid. I was petrified!!

Eventually, Dad stopped and Mum ran out the house wounded and crying. I remember as if it were only yesterday. I rushed out through the front door after her, dropping my teddy Rupert on the way. I was begging her to wait for me as I ran down the street in my nightwear and bare feet.

"Mummy, Mummy! Wait for me!!"

It was a very traumatic experience for me to witness so young. I was only seven. I should have been in bed fast asleep, dreaming lovely dreams. But I was awake. Wide awake and in a living nightmare!

That night Mummy and I walked about a mile to my Grandparents' house. Mummy didn't want to knock on the door and wake them. She said we would have to sleep in the conservatory on the deck chairs. But I found that to be too scary. The wind blowing against the trees in the moonlight made them look like big monsters! So we slept in Granddad's car. Luckily, he hadn't locked the garage door or the car doors. Mum put Granddad's leather driving gloves on my feet to keep me warm. I told Mummy that they looked like monkey's feet. We both laughed for the first time that night.

Mum was pregnant again with my little sister. She considered aborting her as Dad's violence was getting worse! She couldn't take the stress!

It was the last straw for Mum the night Dad put a gun to her head threatening to kill her, then us kids, and then her parents.

Mum had got to the point where enough was enough! So, she left, taking my baby sister and one of my older sisters, leaving me and my other older sister to live with Daddy.

Despite me still having my eldest sister and my father in my life, I still remember feeling very insecure, lost and confused. I was a shadow of my former self. I didn't know who I was! Though Daddy was treating me ok, I was missing Mummy!

It was all very odd and painful for me to cope with all of this at such a young age!

I still attended infant school every day. At least that was the one thing that was consistent in my life. I was happy there. I felt safe there too. And the teachers were really nice! Little did I know that the school I loved and the friends I adored were to come to an abrupt end, which would have a serious negative effect on my life.

I wasn't expecting to see Mummy waiting outside the school gates as I was leaving one day. It was the first time I had seen her since she left us. However, my heart was breaking when she led me up the street in the opposite direction of where "home" was. She told me that we couldn't go back to Daddy and that we were going to live in a new house with her friend and her daughter and my sisters. I had never met this particular friend of hers ever. I didn't want to go. I felt very anxious about this. I felt angry and sad too! I cried out to Mummy. I pulled hard on her hand and tried to stop her from taking me away from Daddy. He and I had got closer since Mummy went away. I loved him! I loved her! I wanted to go home and for Mummy and my sisters to come back home too! But she wasn't listening to me. I was crying my eyes out. I tried to tell her that I needed to say goodbye to Daddy and to get all my toys and my bear Rupert. But it seemed that all I said was in vain. It seemed that she didn't care about how I was feeling or what I needed. All Mum could say was, "Hush now Amy Jean. We are going to live in a new house, and that's that!"

It was odd living in this new house. It felt alien to me. I tried to talk to Mummy. She wasn't listening to me. I felt alone. She and her friend were having lots of parties there. Lots of strangers coming and going. I felt insecure. I wanted to go home and see Daddy! But I didn't see him for a very long time. I couldn't sleep. I felt sad! I found this change very hard to cope with.

I was nine. We moved into a new house. It seemed ok. But Mummy had different boyfriends. One was an Italian man. He loved to fuss my little sister. She got lots of attention. He just patted me on the head like I was a dog. I felt I didn't fit in. I felt angry! I didn't feel happy!

Mummy had a new husband. I was ten. I called him Daddy. He seemed nice. I grew to love him. Mummy worked two jobs now, and was hardly home. Often I had to look after my little sister. She was naughty sometimes. I smacked her. She told Mummy, then Mummy punished me severely and I was sent to bed without supper. I only smacked my sister because I had learnt that from Mummy. I was only a child myself. I didn't know what to do!

I was twelve. I started secondary school. I was being bullied a lot. It was bad! I hated school. I tried to do my work. I was good at it, especially art. But I couldn't concentrate. When I got home, my new Daddy started to hurt me: physically and then sexually. I tried to tell Mummy, but she wasn't listening

I came home one day in tears. I had been attacked by a gang of girls. I lost my coat my new Daddy had bought me. I was traumatised. The bullies did some nasty things to me. I was in pain. Mummy was still at work when I got home. My new Daddy was there. He was in the kitchen. He was angry with me for losing my coat. He beat me. I was screaming in pain. It hurt so much! My little sister saw it! She was crying! He stopped beating me. My sister and I then ran and hid under the stairs until Mummy came home. I showed her the bright red hand marks on me. I told her I was sick from the pain. She tutted, then just told me to be a good girl, then my new Daddy wouldn't hurt me. I told her that he was rubbing his penis against me when he walked by me. She wasn't listening to me. She told me that I was exaggerating. She stayed with him another three years. The abuse got worse! But I was too afraid to tell Mummy. She wouldn't believe me. She wouldn't do anything. My new

Daddy told me that she would hate me if I told on him and that she would send me away to a home! I didn't want to upset Mummy. I wanted her to love me! So I kept silent.

I ran away. I was fifteen. I went to Stratford.

I walked around for hours, wishing I could knock on somebody's door and ask them to help me! But I didn't, because I was too anxious. I kept walking. It got very dark. I was feeling afraid and insecure. I went to a phone box. I tried to sleep but I was crying! I phoned my older sister. I asked her to help me.

My sister and her husband came to pick me up. I lived with them for a while. They were really good to me. They listened to me. They helped me. Though I was very grateful, I felt uncomfortable after a while because they hadn't been married that long and I didn't want to be a burden. They didn't need my problems. I left, and went back home.

Thankfully my stepfather had gone!

Mummy had changed. She was a lot harder! I think all she went through had caused that. As adult now, and as a mother myself, I can appreciate how the stress of volatile relationships can have a huge negative and damaging impact on one's personality and can consequently cause insecurity and pain within the family structure. But as a child, despite what my mother was going through, I still needed her to care about me. I needed her to listen to me. I was desperate for her to show some compassion and to understand what I was going through.

Though I tried to reach out to her, to gain her love and support, she ignored me and cuddled up with my little sister on the sofa! I remember it well, as if it were yesterday. It hurts me still that Mummy was more interested in a TV show than my inner pain!

My first really noticeable mood swing was strong! I threatened to smash all of Mum's bone china on her Welsh dresser. I was also crying my eyes out really hard, as I continued to beg her to listen. I was desperate to do anything to get her attention. However, Mummy continued to ignore me. All she could say was, "Just shut up and go to bed!!"

I took my first overdose. I was still only fifteen! Despite me trying to kill myself, Mummy still didn't listen to me. She was cross that I tried to kill myself. She scolded me for it. I couldn't understand why Mummy favoured my little sister. But then, I knew deep inside that I was a reminder of when Daddy was too violent to her. I was the reason she had to stay with Daddy for seven more years, to take his drunken beatings. I felt Mummy didn't want me. When Mummy was cross or angry with me, and especially when drunk... she would sometimes say, in a harsh voice, through pursed lips, "Oh, my God! You look just like your father!! And then she would add, "You're a mistake anyway! You should never have been born!"

I couldn't cope. Mummy had so many boyfriends coming to the house. I didn't like it. It made me nervous! Some of them paid attention to me that I didn't like. One of them, who was more of a lodger, who seemed ok and was nice to me, asked Mummy if he could take me out to dinner to a posh restaurant to celebrate my sixteenth birthday. He was to pick me up after my performance at the Belgrade Theatre (in Coventry) where I was acting in a play as part of the Belgrade Youth Theatre. (I liked acting. It was an escape for me to be somebody else for a while. I felt safe in another character.) He picked me up in a flashy white TR7 Sports convertible. He was not a particularly nice-looking man, but he was dressed up really smart. My fellow acting friends were excited for me to be going out somewhere nice. They waved me goodbye. I asked this man where Mummy was. He told me she was busy! It was just him and me. I was not happy. But I wanted to go. I was still on a high from the performance. I had never been to a posh restaurant before. We went to a French restaurant in Stratford. He kept giving me wine. I felt drunk. I didn't usually drink alcohol. On the drive home I felt faint. I passed out. I woke up, he was inside me. I was screaming! He was raping me!

He drove me home. Mummy chased him out of the house with a carving knife, telling him to never return! I felt dirty! I bathed often. I scrubbed my skin hard with a scrubbing brush to make myself clean. I did it hard. My skin bled! I had dreamt that one day I would lose my virginity to a man I would fall in love with. Somebody very special. But now that could never ever happen. I was soiled.

I ran away again. I got a job as a Nanny for a friend of the family. I lived there. It was just the man. His wife had left. He came to my room and abused me. I ran away again! I was nearly seventeen. I got a live-in job in a hotel in Nottingham. I put on a brave face in the interview. I acted as if I were really tough and positive! But really, inside myself...I was lost, insecure and very afraid. During my time of work there, my persona kept changing. Mood swings of highs and terrible lows! The manager noticed this. He had no sympathy. I lost my job.

I managed to find other work and accommodation and got involved with a man who took advantage of my weaknesses.

I ran away. I went back to my Mum. She was reluctant to have me there and made me feel uncomfortable. I embarked on a work program course with YOP (Youth Opportunities Program). I met a man, my new boyfriend. We fell in love. I felt happy! He was older than me, a lot older, but he loved me. I was eighteen. I fell pregnant with him. I was over the moon. Delighted I would soon have a baby to love and cherish. But how would I tell Mum?

She was very angry with me. Disappointed in me. She folded her arms. She was frowning at me. "What!?? That's awful!! You must get rid of it, right away!!"

I was horrified by what she was saying!

"No, NO! I can't Mummy!! I can't kill my baby! I want to keep my baby. It's mine!!"

Mummy wasn't listening. She didn't care! She was cold and her face had that hard expression on it, just like it did when she made me kill my pet mouse, Suki.

"If you don't get rid of it, you will have to go!!"

I told my boyfriend. I knew he would be happy! He would let me go and live with him somewhere. We would raise the baby together. We would be a family!

He was furious with me. He ganged up with Mummy. I sat there crying my heart out. They were telling me I must abort it for its own good.

"I don't want a baby!" he said. "I already have three from my previous marriage. If you keep it I will leave you!"

Mummy looked on with her cold stern expression.

I felt lost, alone, terrified!! What was to become of me! I couldn't have a baby on the streets!! I had no savings or chance of a job! Who would employ me, if I was with child?

I didn't realise that my issues with Mental Health had already really begun. In fact, probably from childhood. But nobody noticed. This bad treatment from my Mum and my boyfriend just pushed me further into depression. I was so low. So scared of being kicked out.

The day of the abortion will haunt me for the rest of my life! Not only did it kill my unborn child. It killed a huge part of me!! I was never to be the same ever again! The loss of my unborn child haunts me daily, and it will for the rest of my life!

Not long after I had to give up my baby, due to the threats of my Mum kicking me out, I slipped more and more into depression. I did go away to stay with an auntie of mine, who has been my rock ever since. She tried to help me recover. But sadly I became anorexic, bulimic. I wanted the earth to swallow me up! I had a complete mental breakdown.

I was about twenty when I was finally admitted and sectioned. It was in a psychiatric hospital where sadly my nightmare continued: I had to endure some harrowing things, such as being held down by two nurses while another nurse shoved roast beef into my mouth. I was a vegetarian and I was anorexic! This was so horrific. The Psychiatrist also dangled a carrot in front of me, promising me that I could go home for a weekend if I had a course of ECT treatment. Being wired up to electrics terrified me. But I wanted to go home! I reluctantly signed the paperwork. If I could turn back the clock to that day, I would not have signed. I have been left with life long side effects that I cannot do anything about, which breaks my heart.

Another horrific and traumatic experience for me during my admission there was having to endure the terrifying ordeal of being drugged up to the eyeballs by a male nurse who worked the night shift and drug duty. Night after night I was to be subjected to him sexually abusing me. It was hell on Earth for me. The awful thing, also, was when I tried to tell other staff about it they just put it down to me hallucinating due to my illness at the time, and the memory of my past child abuse. I even tried to tell my mum, but she didn't believe me either. This was one of my first experiences of stigma. Nobody listened to me. They just blamed the illness. So sad. So very wrong!!

The mental and emotional scars of that awful abuse I endured in Psychiatric Hospital haunts me still, and often. This experience, amongst others, has had a significant negative effect on my relationships. I find it hard to trust.

I believe that this is because of all I went through as a child, including the abuse and the day Mummy made me kill my pet mouse and another pet my daddy had bought me to make me feel better after Suki died - my beautiful guinea pig Guinevere , whom she let freeze to death in the cold winter, despite me begging her to let me bring her into the warmth in a corner of our huge kitchen. And the fact that she pressured me to abort my little child growing inside my womb, with its little heart already ticking away. A life. My baby!! These things would be enough in themselves. Then there were the sexual abuse and the bullying. Also the breakup of my Mum's two marriages, both at difficult ages for me. The first being when she left Daddy, when I was only seven. Then the sudden change when I ran away at fifteen, during my mock exams. I never did go back to school. I left there without saying farewell to my friends. Though I was glad to see the back of the bullies, and my stepfather ...

It was all too much trauma for me as a child and teenager to endure. Growing up is difficult enough to cope with!

Even though I did manage to form some sort of life after having gone through a lot of hell in my early life, sadly the consequences of my experiences formed me into who I became for the rest of my adult life. I am insecure, fragile at times. I let people walk all over me.

Even the abuse continued, due to me falling for the wrong guys. And I always forgave them for what they did to me! For some reason I seemed to go for men who reminded me of my father, which is crazy, really. He drank a lot, and was extremely violent! In all honesty, I think I found some comfort in those sorts of relationships, as they were familiar to me. This pattern in my life continued right through, until only a few years ago, in relationships with men.

I have tried several times to end my life even up to the present time. Just a few days ago, I wanted to throw myself off the bridge over the ring road, as I cycled across it. I wanted to turn all the pain off that still has a tight grip on my very soul! It seems the only way to escape from the dark memories that haunt me every day.

I also can't deal with the stigma attached to my mental health issues. Many members of my family, even my own mother and father, when they were alive, treated me differently, as if I was crazy. It was so soul-destroying. Also, sadly, some of my siblings and other members of my family and some friends see me as odd and do their best to avoid me, due to the stigma. And some have even said that they make excuses for my mood swings and persona issues because they say it's not my fault, and that I am just crazy!! This really upsets me. Because I am not "crazy!" I am a human being who was born into a violent, dysfunctional family and suffered so terribly from other things too in my early life, and beyond. I feel like I am like an autumn leaf being tossed about in the wind. Helpless!

I have managed to hold a few jobs down in the past, despite having had some grief from fellow workers taking advantage of my health issues. I also saw a college course right through and obtained an international Qualification in Remedial Therapy. Sadly though, getting a job is extremely difficult due to difficulties arising from a physical disability also: Functional Movement Disorder - a psychosomatic illness, which the neurologist said has been possibly brought on from past trauma. Also, my bike accident hasn't helped as I had a hard knock to the head which the specialist said probably caused a glitch in the software of my brain. MS-like symptoms, but not hard-drive causes, so to speak. This, alongside my Mental Health issues, has worked very much against me.

Believe me, I have tried. I applied for a post as a remedial therapist at the Walsgrave University Hospital, in Coventry, a few years ago. I had to be honest about my mental health issues, as there is a section on the application form that one has to fill in. I was honest. I never got a response back. I didn't get even an interview!

Yet despite every awful thing I have been through, and endure to this very day, I did experience some happiness on my journey of development and pain, including: living in South Wales with an auntie, uncle and cousins, enjoying the beautiful countryside and attending school there, where I did make new friends also. As well as that, I did have some really nice times with my mother and father and my siblings too! It wasn't all doom and gloom. Though I was still a wide-eyed bewildered and damaged child, I carried on as best as I could.

Despite my marriage failing, I am a very fortunate

woman in the sense that I was blessed to be a mother to my wonderful son whom I love with all of my heart and soul! It hasn't been easy for him, either. He, too, suffers with depression. He, too, is a victim of witnessing violence from childhood when his stepfather was physically violent to me and to him also. It got that bad at one time that my son was taken from me, and spent time in foster care, which has left some emotional scars with him and me. Despite the violence from my son's stepfather it was very hard to leave him, as he threatened to kill both me and my son if we did.

Among other difficult experiences, my son also had to try to cope growing up with me and struggling to understand and deal with my mental health issues. It has been extremely difficult for him. But love has got us through! We have a good mother and son relationship that goes from strength to strength and that is a blessing for sure!

My son and I not only have a strong bond: we are both determined to help each other make a difference in this world to help bring about positive change in removing the stigma from mental health issues once and for all. We don't want anybody else to suffer the way we have. We want to help them have a voice! Somehow, some way!

It has been a blessing and an honour to have been

invited to tell my story of how mental health issues and stigma have affected my life, and my son's. And though extremely painful for me at times to write, it has been a cathartic journey. Thank you to the members of my family and to the friends who played a part in doing their best to help support us through these difficult times. Thank you also to a friend who made a positive difference in my life by giving me a box of art materials and encouraging me to paint! Having the opportunity to express my pain through art is helping in the healing process. I also want to say a huge Thank You to Polly Fielding for having invited me to write my story. Without you, Polly, I wouldn't have had a voice! And finally, I would like to say thank you to all who have purchased and read this book. You have made a difference.

Bless you. I hope that it can help you and others in some way, for the better! My best wishes to you all.

Lauren's Story

For as long as I can remember I always knew I was different. Growing up I had an awful childhood. I lived in a house that was constantly abusive. I was hit around with sticks, slippers, belt, sand, fists. I was verbally abused, being called fat, ugly, stupid and useless. I was constantly told that nobody would like me and I was not good enough to be anybody or anything. I used to have a lock on the outside of my bedroom door where I would often be locked in. Some nights I would have the handles taken off my door so I was unable to seek comfort from my brother who, being a lot younger, did not experience any of this. As a teenager I lived in my room and I sought comfort from self-harming - using a compass to cut at my arms.

I was very quiet and shy and had very few friends. I used to cling to teachers or older people that I felt safe with. This caused me to create a bubble in my head and it's where I felt safe. While at high school, I adored a teacher and she became like my mother. I used to dream of what it would be like living with her and having that mother I could talk to and go shopping with. Most importantly somebody who loved me as a daughter. It broke my heart to not be able to have that, especially after I heard them talking about the things they did as a family. I never had many new clothes and when I was fifteen I had to find a weekend job to be able to live at home and they took all my money. On top of this I was sexually abused and at nineteen I was raped.

I was unable to hold down any jobs as I was so paranoid that people hated me and my confidence and self esteem were non-existent. I couldn't talk to people, I had no friends and relationships completely broke down. I had my first child at eighteen, due to being left to fend for myself. I then had my other child at twenty-four and that relationship broke down due to me being clingy and him having an affair while I was twelve weeks pregnant. By this time I was trying to stay strong. However, a year after my daughter was born, it was noticed by somebody that I had depression. I denied this fact as I thought it was me. As I always felt different I was unable to see what the problem was.

In 2008, I attended a church service where something strange happened. I just completely broke down. It was the most distressing and confusing time and the worst was yet to come. I became so withdrawn that I was unable to connect properly with my children. I started drinking quite a lot along with sleeping around and self-harming. I just wanted somebody to help me, to love me, to like me. In 2011, I became pregnant with my little boy. I became really unwell and after the birth in 2012, I became severely depressed. I would sit in the house and not go out. I cried constantly and I was unable to bond with the baby. He cried a lot and in turn I would scream at him, and most nights I would be sat on the stairs rocking back and forth. I turned back to alcohol to help, but instead of it helping, I became more detached and unwell and in turn became severely suicidal. I would text the few older mother figures I made friends with, telling them how I couldn't live anymore and I wanted to kill myself.

It was in August 2012 that I took an overdose and tried to kill myself. It was only because I had been texting a friend and told her what I planned to do and that I had done it, that she came down and saved me. After this point, I lost contact with the few mother figures I had. This made me feel more suicidal as I couldn't see why they were abandoning me, especially after what I had been through. I remember one friend saying to me that all my texting of not being able to cope and suicide was too upsetting and she couldn't talk to me until I was better. Another said, "There is nothing wrong with you. It's your fault you're in this mess." My good friend would turn her phone off and ignore my cries for help. I was unable to understand what was wrong with me. It was so frightening.

I began ten weeks of CBT (Cognitive Behaviour Therapy) in January 2013. However, my Occupational Therapist realised this was not working and agreed to keep seeing me until she could get the right treatment I needed. In the meantime, I was still cutting and researching ways to commit suicide. I would find comfort in reading suicidal quotes and planning my funeral. I did have relapses in putting light cords around my neck to ease how I felt and it worked. After eighteen months of regularly seeing my OT (Occupational Therapist), I was introduced to a consultant psychologist who specialises and trains professionals in DBT (also known as Dialectical Behavioural Therapy). I began my treatment in May 2014 where I had individual therapy and in September 2014 I began the group skills training with another nine patients. Having therapy twice a week, along with homework and phone coaching, was very tough and extremely emotional. However, I have found it to be the best treatment around. It covers skills in:

Mindfulness

Distress Tolerance

Emotional Regulation

Interpersonal Effectiveness

I have learnt so much and in December 2014 I was finally given a Diagnosis of BPD (Borderline Personality Disorder) and Complex Trauma.

To fight for a diagnosis was hard as professionals are extremely reluctant in diagnosing people with mental illness. This was very concerning and stigmatising, as I believe every individual has the right to a diagnosis, just like cancer patients, so they are able to access the correct treatment.

Researching about BPD I became very much aware that even mental health professionals are very ignorant towards patients like myself and other BPD sufferers. According to them we are manipulative, attention seeking and extremely hard work and this type of illness is not serious. I have a few peers who have been admitted within the past three months, and as soon as these professionals have read their notes, they have been ignored and unspoken to. I have recently completed my first six months in DBT and I am now completing my last six months. In this time I have made a great group of friends who understand me and we have our own facebook page where we are able to talk about anything that is bothering us. I am able to label and notice my emotions and feelings and I am learning a lot through mindfulness.

My major achievement is I have completely stopped all impulsive behaviours such as self-harm and suicide. I don't look up suicide anymore and I am hoping to start voluntary work on the mental health ward shadowing an OT. I have also been training with my psychologist and attended mindfulness groups. In the next six months I am hoping to become a DBT Peer Support Mentor.

I believe this treatment along with mindfulness has been my lifeline. I don't believe I would be here today if I did not access this treatment.

The Government needs to give the NHS more funding within the mental health department, so that this therapy can become widely available and help save more lives.

Kil's Story

So fresh in my memory. The house – a decaying body, my family – the bile being pushed around, until our inevitable exit came from the excretion of this hell. Daddy wasn't living with us anymore, but he was living in our fears, at least. This new house was meant to be a new beginning, say goodbye to the past with a smile. Tomorrow will be okay. Every night – in actuality, the early hours of the morning – he would drag his feet to our front door – drunk, high, who knows? – banging and shouting, threatening and terrifying. He was my father, once upon a time but that time is gone. All that remains are the memories that imitate God, and so it continues... the haunting of a ghost still very much alive...

My younger brother was tiny, my older brother was bigger and there was me in the middle, age was not important. The past wasn't important. The future wasn't important. Who we were or who we'd subsequently become wasn't important either. All that mattered was the there and now. What if, no matter how rich or poor, good or evil, sane or insane we are, we all end up in the same place after death? We'd all be equal in the dread or bliss – whichever way you look at all – of nothingness. What then, would that mean for my life? Daddy was always a scary kind of person, whenever we'd hear him and mummy arguing, he would sound like the personification of hell, a volcano in the abyss, ready to erupt. Things would go flying, chairs, tables, TVs through closed, now broken windows and there was always the fear that one of these days we'd all end up dead...

I remember once he got the belt – or at least, my memory tells me it was a belt – and he whacked me and my older brother with it. Just a short, stark memory and then it's gone. Another one, we're standing by the front door of the first home I ever lived in: I remember the dullness and the yellow light. I remember feeling so small. It must've been 1997 because I'm pretty sure my little brother was about one. Daddy had been in the middle of the ten millionth argument with mummy when he'd threatened to kill my little brother – that sticks in my head. Spiteful? I think it's safe to class that as an understatement. We lived in fear, and fear led to a shared depression. But we all dealt with it differently. Mine turned inward and I've never really felt like there was anyone who could truly help... except maybe death?

At school, I was never really bullied and I got on with most people, yet there was always something that made me feel miserable...

Of course, in hindsight a lot of things have become clearer, and certain incidents, like when daddy was driving me home but then stopped outside of some... place, to meet some... woman. With the lack of innocence adults grow into, it's clearer than ever as to what was going on. I remember seeing a mobile on the seat as I waited in the back of daddy's car, waiting for ages to go home, and so I rung mummy and told her what was going on... not because I wanted to grass daddy up, I didn't know he was doing anything wrong; but mummy did and she came, there was a bit of drama and the rest slips from my memory.

The only piece of advice, or 'wisdom' from daddy that I remember receiving... was something along the lines of, 'When you grow older, you'll understand that men can't stay faithful' and 'Watch out for any black girls; they might be related to you'. Those words didn't make sense until majority hit and innocence died. Daddy was telling us that he was a whore and according to him, that is Man's inherited shame.

Something, deeper inside of my psyche kept me miserable, even when I should really be happy. Am I insane? Maybe I'm an alien. Do they know? Paranoia.

There's little bits and pieces of life between then

and the end of his reign as 'Father' to us that could be included in this cognitive journey back in time, but to condense it and put it in a jar of flies, all one needs to say is, what he was, is everything I don't want to be. If I was ever going to smoke weed, I wouldn't. If I was ever going to rely on alcohol to quench my thirst, I wouldn't, if I was ever going to smoke, I wouldn't, if I ever was going to destroy what I helped create, I wouldn't. Maybe it was the nihilistic streak in him that drove him insane, or maybe it was his insanity that triggered the nihilism within; either way, he was destructive and for many years, the greatest thing I felt he destroyed, was me. Broken, depressed, alone, ridiculous, futile, unnecessary, suicidal, bored, confused, breathing yet far from being alive...

Music became my catharsis and bands like Placebo, System of a Down, Nirvana, Our Lady Peace, Staind, Machine Head, Metallica, Death, Opeth, My Dying Bride and Paradise Lost, just to name a few, became my medicine. I decided that I could live, because there was hope. Music gave me something to look forward to, music became my new daddy. I wanted to be a musician, not only to live with great wealth (and health), but to be able to share my angst, my pain, and my vision with the world – that way I felt. Maybe, just maybe, my pain wouldn't have been endured in vain. Maybe I can write songs, lyrics, riffs, concepts, about my inner conflicts and hopefully, not only will it entertain many, but it will act too as a catharsis for those in need. I found creativity as my way out.

But every time I've tried to arise, I seem to fall. So much ambition, so much hope, but then I feel too forlorn and drained to follow through. Back into my bed I go. Every little thing upsets me, turning the news on kills me, I feel ambition-less, I feel alien, I feel drained, I feel like the living dead, breathing yet far from alive... and I know where it comes from, I know where it comes from... and sometimes he'd be there, he'd be driving me and my brothers through burning streets at a deathly speed, or manipulating my mum into some torturous scenario, and then I'd be brought back to life, no longer asleep, awoken by the sounds of mother's screams... and I don't know whether or not I'm relieved to be awake or wish that instead I was still asleep.

A lot of people have asked me, 'Why can't you just be happy?' A lot of people have wondered what's 'wrong' with me, and in turn I've wondered the same thing. Maybe out of curiosity, maybe I'd like to know, just in case, you know... one day I decide to answer one of those questions myself, and I find that the reason I cannot be happy is because happiness despises me. What's wrong with me?

Well, this is my natural response to the fact that happiness does not want me. Rejected. Maybe I'm cursed, maybe I'm just wrong. But then I sleep it off and that side of me – that negative side of me that I've named Dolorosa Tristesse – is now asleep and the more positive side of my nature awakens, and we start over. We can do this, we can make positive of this negative situation. We can make light of this darkness. We can make freedom of this emotional rape. Maybe we can find a job working with children, or depressed people, something that makes you feel useful, something that makes you feel rewarded. But I want to be creative. After all, I studied creative subjects at Uni, I need to be creative or I'll be a failure to my Self...

Oh, the Self, pulled left and right by the Id and the ego, and there's the Self in the middle, staring back at me, wondering which side I'm going to be on today. When there's no balance, everything's confused, my mind splits in two, yet again, now making four, eight and so on, until each piece is a smaller piece of the thing that it once was, now the thing that should not be... and I feel like the living dead, awake and dreaming, breathing, but by no means alive...

I feel the fire burning, but I know it's just a heavy memory, I hear the screams, I hear him shout at me, 'Where's your mum!?' I see myself point him in the wrong direction, I feel the fire, I see his anger, I see the knife and the vicious lunacy in his eyes. I see the rest of my family jump from the window, onto the mattress, across the road and into the neighbours, where I am, watching them. I see them run, I see the neighbour shut the door, I see daddy chasing in, I see him kick the door open with one powerful foot, I see him pounce on mummy and cut her, I see big brother wrestle him off with all his strength, I see myself, the coward who ran downstairs, opened the door and almost put us all in direct danger. I see the fire burning and I see him standing in front of me as I open the door, he's asking me where my mum is?! He's expecting me to tell him, so he can kill her. He's expecting me to tell him, so he can change my life forever. I lie, I send him the wrong way, with that knife in his hand, he comes back, shouting at me, I am a liar. I AM A LIAR! And I see him running down the road when the police finally get here...

I see calm, he's not there yet, but we're all upstairs, in the un-decorated house, something's about to happen, but no one knows that, not yet anyway, only me, because now I'm watching everything with brand new eyes. Eyes which I wish that I could trade because with all that I've been through, and all that I've learned, I know that a new Self has been born. Every suicidal ideation, every dark thought that strays from the realms of 'normal' I will place the blame on him. He will not define who I am. He will not define who I am. He will... he will define who I am. He does define who I am because I hate myself, I hate my life, I hate what I've been through and where I've been. I hate my thoughts, and most of them remain between myself and me. But that's not me, that's Dolorosa, that safe, negative place in my mind that I can visit whenever I need to vent, whenever I need to be a freak without the judgement of another Self. But me... if I am not my arms, my chest, my heart or my brain, then who am I? If I am my mind, then which one am I?

Some days I feel okay, but in some daze I'm completely lost. I'm lost and have no interest in ever returning. I feel that with the curse I'm under, no matter how hard I try, depression, misery and failure will always be a part of me. I feel that no matter what I do, I will be done. And as I write this, I turn to my left, an Anathema CD beside me, 'A Fine Day to Exit', and I wonder as my mind continues to wander... what if?

Bridget's Story

I have been reading lately of how many men are being subjected to spousal abuse from their wives and the shame that they feel, as well as the fear of ridicule from other men if they were to speak about it. I couldn't help wondering, if they were to interview those abusive wives, just how many of them might be suffering from PMT (pre-menstrual tension)?

I ask this because I was once an abuser too and I had no idea that, those few days before my period was due, my raging hormones changed me from a mild-mannered but reasonably laid back wife and mother, into an almost homicidal maniac. I never had any pains or dreadful cramps like a lot of women suffered and no heavy bleeding either. It lasted for only three days exactly and was over until the next month. However, I was in my twenties before I began to connect my foul temper and rages to those few days before my period. I decided to go to my doctor and tell him but was too ashamed to mention that I was actually beginning to try and physically hurt my partner, just told him about my rages and screaming fits. He just smiled condescendingly at me and said not to worry because it was quite a common problem and he would give me some sleeping tablets as I was probably very tired and run down. I actually felt like hitting him as well at the time but I walked out and vowed I would not take sleeping pills ever.

When the 'rages' took over, it was as if I was standing outside of my body, watching me lash out to my partner and listening to the cruel and abusive things I was saying. I wanted to stop, I was hating everything I was doing but I was somehow powerless to do so. I knew there was something seriously wrong with me and I was so ashamed of my behaviour; I tried once more to talk about it to another doctor and this time I told him everything. All the time he did not look at me once and was scribbling on a pad in front of him. When I had finished talking, he looked up and said, "You know, you are very lucky your partner has not left you, or at the very least, hit you back. I think you should count your blessings that he obviously cares for you. I think you need to learn how to calm down and be grateful for him, not many men would stay around in your situation."

From that moment on, I felt so much shame, knowing what he thought of me, and realised that I was not going to get any help or understanding whatsoever. I went home, determined to try and be better but what I began to call my 'insane days' took over completely and eventually he left me, or should I say more truthfully, I threw him out, and he went back to live with his mother again. It was only because I cared for him and was terrified I would really seriously harm him if he stayed with me any longer. I begged him not to tell anyone what I had done to him and his reply was that I was a mental case and he would not want anyone to know that he was being attacked by me anyway, so my secret was safe.

Once more the overwhelming shame filled me, as well as my fear that I was a mental case maybe? Once he had left, my 'insane days' took the form of me shouting at my children and then kicking the hell out of anything in my way. Eventually I met someone else and gradually my rages began to surface again. This time, he persuaded me to go back to my doctor.

Nervous and scared, I turned up for the appointment. He listened to me and after I had told him everything he said, "Well, you obviously have PMT, which thousands of women go through, so you don't have to get too upset about it, it's fairly normal. I will give you some medication, anti-depressants, and this might help. You could of course see a psychiatrist but it's a long wait and once you go along that path, you are going to be regarded as mentally ill and this is just a normal thing for women to go through, so take the medication and see how you go. You will grow out of it eventually."

Once again, I felt stupid and lost and now I had been told that if I did seek out any further help, it would mean I would be totally stigmatised as a mentally ill person. What choice did I have but to take the medication?

Two months later, I abandoned the pills because they made me sleepy and disorientated and my rages still occurred but I hadn't the energy to scream and use physical violence, instead I just harboured hateful thoughts against my partner. Once the pills had come out of my system, it was back to the rages again and a year later, I was so scared that I would kill him that I ran away and left him with my children for two weeks. When I returned, he wouldn't let me back into my home and I spent six months trying to get custody of my children and my home back.

About a year later I met someone else and the same thing happened again. I became pregnant and while I was in hospital, I demanded to be sterilised before I left the hospital and after telling a doctor what I was going through, he felt that it was grounds for me to have it done in case my anger turned towards my children. He also made it obvious what he thought of my behaviour and stated that was the only reason that he would perform the sterilisation. Arrangements were made for the op to be done that afternoon and then I returned home the next day.

It was about three months later that I noticed I had not felt anything at all on my 'rage days' and I went through each month with no change at all in my behaviour. After a year, I realised that whatever changes the sterilisation had made to my body, it had changed my mental status, too.

The PMT never returned but it was no thanks to the doctors who should have helped me. Instead, all they ever did was to compound my fears that I was a 'mental case' and it was my fault, as if I actually chose to be violent and that I should pull myself together because it was my fault, not my imbalanced hormones.

I will never be able to forget what happened and how it almost destroyed my life, as well as the pain and violence I inflicted on my ex-partners. Thank God that I insisted on that operation because I know for sure that I was capable of killing someone and so very close to going over the edge then. The overriding anger that I felt, and still feel, towards the doctors, was not because of their lack of proper treatment und understanding but because I was made to feel even more guilty than I already did and because of the terrifying fear of being a mental case for the rest of my life.

My heart goes out to those women who suffer from this terrible affliction. Even after so many years, there is still little sympathy or understanding of this mental illness. I wonder just how many of these women are going through hell, unable or afraid to seek help because of this and the only way we know about it is when we see the headlines in the media after they have killed, or attempted to kill, their partners. It could so easily have been me but why do I still keep it hidden, still feel ashamed of what happened? I am just as guilty of perpetuating the secrecy and the shame. Maybe one day it might get better but we have a long way to go before that happens.

Alma's Story

From Both Sides

I've enjoyed listening to the Joni Mitchell song 'I've looked at love from both sides now' many times. As I sit down to put my story on paper, it seems an appropriate way to sum up my experience of Mental Illness and the assumptions I've encountered around my own mental health and diagnosis.

For ten years I worked as a Probation Officer with a significant proportion of my caseload being Mentally Disordered Offenders (MDOs). At the time the Probation Service still existed as a statutory public body and we worked in multi-agency teams to manage the most dangerous and prolific offenders. Most MDOs who, it seemed to me, were essentially those designated as being capable of management using medication and under the care of a Psychiatrist, were the only ones deemed worthy of local psychiatric intervention and support. This meant that 'Mental Illness' as defined for intervention by local mental health specialists was very narrow and rarely helped us in managing the most challenging behaviour.

Most of the emotional and mental health issues we

encountered were bundled up in complex human needs, comprising traumatic childhood abuse, self-medication through alcohol and illegal substances and many offenders who had been victims of violence. Many of my MDOs, if they had diagnoses, were designated as suffering symptoms of 'Personality Disorder'. This was a 'get out of jail free' card for the local psychiatric teams up until 2007 as until then, such a diagnosis had the label of 'untreatable'. Most multi-agency meetings, aimed at finding the best way of managing such offenders for the safety of both the public and the individuals themselves, ended with the words from (usually) the psychiatrist stating, 'Untreatable, this is a Criminal Justice problem.' Along with my Police colleagues, I was constantly frustrated and ended up working as counsellor and emergency contact as such people had been banned from local A&E departments, due to their behaviour towards others when emotionally distressed. Recently, there has been an acknowledgement that police holding cells and standard prison regimes are not appropriate settings in which to contain and address mental health related offending and presentation.

In 2007 the Mental Health Act sought to establish Personality Disorder as a diagnosis with a treatment pathway. This coincided with a deterioration in my own mental health and finally an assessment and diagnosis of Borderline Personality Disorder (BPD) in 2009.

Most people dislike the diagnosis of BPD because it essentially labels the whole person as being 'defective'. For me, terms like 'emotionally sensitive', or 'emotionally dysregulated' are more helpful in some ways, except they fail to capture the all-pervasive nature of the emotional and psychological distress experienced by me. So I'm left with BPD as a label that works for me as a shorthand when people ask me what my 'problem' is.

I was only diagnosed in my early forties, having been treated on and off for 'stress related' breakdowns associated with Clinical Depression all my life. Having had my first encounter with mental health services in school, aged sixteen, I considered myself as someone who was susceptible to depression. No one managed to ask any questions that opened up symptoms around suicidal feelings and self harm, so I kept that 'sort of thing' to myself. Besides, usually after about six to nine months on an anti-depressant I would 'recover' and literally restart my life. Different location, different career, brand new relationships (because as part of my 'depressive episodes' I would have burnt all my bridges). Such constant uprooting, lack of stability in relationships and loss of identity evident in these periods of breakdown, are key symptoms of BPD. Yet, no one, from a Consultant Psychiatrist to Rape Counsellors ever completed a full life and psychiatric history with me, until 2009. I had had my first mental health referral at school in 1982.

When I was finally diagnosed with BPD in 2009 I was relieved. The patterns of collapse and recovery had quite literally left me burnt out and bereft of all sense of who I was, with no sense of being able to experience emotion of any kind. In trying to capture how low I was my GP told me that not only had I run out of 'fuel' and was 'low on energy', she felt I was effectively like a car with no engine. During this time she increased and changed my anti-depressants on three occasions. I was referred to the Graduate Mental Health worker at the practice once again, as my presentation suggested clinical Depression and Stress related illness. To her credit, she quickly discerned that six weeks of brief CBT was not going to touch the issues she had brought out as she asked strategic questions and then, listened. My GP, too, listened, not just to what my symptoms were, but how I felt I was being affected as a person by my emotional and mental turmoil. My mantra at this time was 'I am not made for this world', something I had felt all my life. I felt I couldn't make myself heard or understood, I told my GP, 'I am inside my own head, screaming'.

None of this would have been apparent to anyone giving me a cursory glance. When I finally was signed off sick, all my records and case files were up to date and I had not missed any appointments with my offenders. When I came to a stop, it was sudden and complete. I had ceased functioning in any effective way.

Thankfully, the intervention of the Graduate Worker in pushing me forward for assessment by the Community Mental Health Team, paid off when I was assessed by someone who did not take my 'high functionality' at face value. She was my Care Co-ordinator over the five years from diagnosis, through treatment to discharge in 2014. The therapeutic relationship has been crucial to my engagement in treatment and the beginning of my road to recovery. Because of the chain of care I experienced my view of my diagnosis has been largely positive. I know that for many people with BPD this level of continuity and understanding has not been there and so they have experienced the diagnosis negatively. I know I have been blessed by the quality of care I have received.

Having experienced BPD as a professional and witnessed first-hand the attitudes of many professionals who had failed to see the individuals beyond the challenging behaviours, I was fearful of being labelled unfairly. Looking back I can see that there were times when working with me could have been challenging. Those who managed to work effectively in helping me manage my condition, were the people who asked the question: 'What is it that has created such levels of distress in this person?' and, 'Is this person able to identify and manage their emotions effectively?'

Due to a series of factors I had learned (usually the hard way) about feelings and how the average person expressed these. As someone with BPD, social interaction is not a natural ability. As a young child in my first years at primary school I was selectively mute. I have always struggled to recognise and identify specific feelings in others and myself. I have had to learn to censor myself and use thinking to mask my emotional turmoil. Obviously, there have been ways I have used to manage my emotional distress which have not been effective or helpful to me. From the point of diagnosis I had to learn that this was the case, that though my coping mechanisms had been 'effective' in that I managed to lead an outwardly successful life, ultimately I ended up broken, exhausted and unable to function.

'Treating someone with borderline personality disorder can be one of the toughest challenges a [social worker] encounters. Life for such a client is like trying to drive a car that is constantly careening out of control. Emotional vulnerability, fear of abandonment, and a seemingly invalid environment push the car from one side of the road to the other. The tiniest stressors can force the car into a ditch.'

Quote from: Dialectical Behavior Therapy — Treating Borderline Personality Disorder. By Christina Olenchek, Social Work Today Vol. 8 No. 6 P. 22

If I may borrow from the quote above, anyone observing the 'car' of my life would have seen significant progress. Success in life, even. I had achieved academically, I was successful at sports, managed to hold down highly responsible and well paid jobs, for significant periods of time. However, look closer at the 'driver' and any casual observer would see a panic stricken, emotional wreck, as I struggled to keep my 'car' from careering from one cliff face precipice to the other. My life had developed into a pattern of emotional collapse, exhaustion and recovery, which resulted in my resigning jobs, selling houses and usually prompted the dissolution of my relationships. Every five years or so due to my inability to keep going, I would dismantle my whole life, pack up and move to another area, retrain, usually in another challenging career and rebuild my social life. I did this three or four times from the age of eighteen until I ground to a halt in my forties and found myself unable to do so again.

As I learned more about BPD and particularly the research and therapy of Marsha Linehan, who developed Dialectical Behaviour Therapy (DBT), I came across a phenomenon known as 'apparent competence'. This relates to the 'Swan Effect' where on the surface it was not obvious I was struggling with life, while underneath I was frantically trying to keep myself going, paddling wildly against the waves of emotional distress which threatened to drag me under.

I think the issues around 'apparent competence' are examples of one side of Mental Health stigma which is not often discussed. For those of us, and there are many, who continue to work and function well whilst struggling against complex mental health issues, there is an assumption from Mental Health Services that we are not priorities. After all, we're doing 'okay'. However, as I've pointed out earlier, this ignores the fact that before the 'car' of our life crashes over the precipice we probably were in need of intervention. Unfortunately, for many it takes us to get to the point of suicide or complete emotional and mental collapse before anyone steps in and offers support.

Having had the diagnosis and accepted for myself that I had been suffering the symptoms of BPD from as far back as I remember, I had an immediate decision to make. Given the levels of responsibility entailed in my job, as well as the emotional cost of managing difficult people, I felt that it was important to be honest with my employer about my diagnosis. This proved to be a double-edged sword.

On the day I received my diagnosis, I sat in my car, dumbstruck, wondering whether to just continue on to work, or if there was suddenly some seismic shift in me since I set out for my assessment appointment that morning that would be obvious the minute I walked through the door. As if suddenly, 'Unclean' might have appeared across my forehead.

At the time, my Line Manager was aware that I might be suffering from increasingly severe bouts of depression. This, though, felt really different; somehow I didn't feel as free to talk about more 'Complex Mental Health Issues' with her and I certainly wasn't sure I was prepared to tell her that they were looking at BPD as a diagnosis. Instinctively, I knew that a label was going to change everything. And this one had a lot of baggage attached - Borderline Personality Disorder (BPD).

Being a creature of habit, I continued on to work and debriefed my Manager, deciding that both she and I were the same people we were the day before.

I also decided to trust in the good sense I respected in her as a colleague working with challenging people. I was right. Together we wondered about the label and what it actually meant in practical terms for my job and me as a person. It is hard to find a good Manager, but when you do, really appreciate them. So hurdle one was over, I had told my employer that not only did I have a Mental Health problem, but it was one that I really was only beginning to learn about for myself. Up until that I had only had an interest in PD (Personality Disorder) as a conscientious professional.

Unfortunately, the procedures in place and the attitude of the Senior Managers in charge of my Probation area were not as compassionate about my diagnosis as the person most responsible for my day to day work. Suddenly, from being 'supportive', the shift in sickness procedures became a focus on whether or not I was a risk to my cases. This shows a shocking lack of understanding of mental illness in general and BPD in particular. The sickness absence procedures themselves were applied as a 'one size fits all' solution to long term sickness, regardless of the intrinsic differences between physical and mental illnesses.

I don't think a Senior Manager would ask of a Cancer sufferer, 'A year ago you told us the 'Chemo' would work, so why have you gone off again and are now telling us that you need Radiotherapy?' Unfortunately, having remained at work for eight months following a difficult period, when my initial treatment failed, I was signed off again in 2011 and I was asked by the Senior Manager why the first treatment I had tried had not worked and, 'What guarantee do we have that the new treatment they are suggesting will work and that you will not be signed off again?'

Now, correct me if I'm wrong, but even the most highly regarded medical training does not include crystal ball reading, I believe that's only on offer at Hogwarts! However such questions betray an underlying suspicion, or even prejudice, about mental illness, and that is: it's all in my head! If you don't fit neatly into the procedures which, again and again I was told, were there to support me to remain in work, then employers seem to waver between wanting to help and threatening me with capability procedures. In the end it became impossible for me to remain in work, even on a part-time basis, and engage in the intensive Dialectical Behaviour Therapy programme I was offered a place on.

So can such Sickness Absence procedures deal with the paradox of the worker with mental illness whose work is characterised as 'excellent'? In the present climate the pressure not to disclose mental health issues will grow, but how can we educate employers to view those with mental health problems in the same way that they view physical health problems? With the same level of compassion and support? I was most disappointed because we were a profession trained in risk assessment and management. We learned about the interaction and importance of mental health with drugs and other substances in increasing risk to both the individual and wider community. If my colleagues and senior managers exhibited such limited understanding of Mental Illness and the risks associated with it, what hope did I have of acceptance from the wider community?

Again and again, I was referred to Occupational Health with the same questions: Was I safe to be left alone with violent offenders? What impact was I likely to have on my colleagues? Again, and again Occupational Health staff asked for assessments and reports from those treating me. Again and again, the response came back that my risk was primarily from suicide and that continuing in work was important in providing me with the stability and structure I needed. It sounds ridiculous seeing it in black and white, given that I had worked happily and effectively for the same team for nearly seven years. Amazing that, suddenly, I was the risk to be assessed rather than be the assessor of risk which was one of my main roles at the time. Finally, they decided that they needed to pay for a private Psychiatrist (somehow all the assessments and support being given to me by the NHS had become suspect as they were all emphasising that my risk to others was minimal!). He fudged the issue by asking me my opinion! Again, Apparent Competence meant that even after charging my employers for two one hour assessments during which he demurred on the diagnosis of BPD, he suggested a change in anti-depressant medication and confirmed that I posed no danger to anyone but myself. I decided that the combined experience, observation and assessment of five NHS professionals who had worked with me over a period of eighteen months to arrive at my diagnosis, outweighed the arguably biased view of one privately funded specialist who knew little about me.

In the end, a combination of the ongoing process of referral for risk assessment and scrutiny every time I experienced a dip in mood and worsening of my symptoms, forced me to accept an offer of voluntary redundancy. I think this kind of treatment by employers goes on without challenge simply because the cost of standing up for yourself, along with dealing with your mental illness, is just too difficult to contemplate at the time.

A diagnosis of mental illness is isolating. Suddenly, you're not sure who and what to tell. Every conversation becomes a risk. For me it has been painful at times to realise that some friendships, which have lasted a long time, foundered when my problems had a definition and a way forward. Although there are problems with the diagnosis and the label, it opened up hope that I could overcome it with effective therapies. One of the most helpful moments was my first meeting with my main individual DBT therapist who told me 'I can help you.' For so many who suffer from Mental Illness this, along with the acknowledgement that 'I know you don't want to feel this way', are like beacons of light in the darkness.

From friends, I've had various responses from 'Rubbish, you're just depressed'... (the fact that they can say, 'just' depressed alone, gives an idea of the misunderstanding out there of the impact of mental illness), to 'don't be ridiculous, you've got your own house, car, job'... to 'but you're so normal!'. These responses show out and out ignorance of what Mental Illness is and who can suffer from it.

More subtle have been the responses which initially seemed supportive. But as time went on and they realised that not only was I seeing a CPN monthly, seeing my GP monthly, but I was also expected to attend twice a week for treatment at my local

Mental Health unit, they started to tell me that it was silly the amount of time being taken to 'help' me. After all I had managed for over thirty years without this level of intervention. I guess these reactions demonstrate how far I had managed to mask the worst of my symptoms from those around me. By the time I was diagnosed, no one in my life at the time was aware that I frequently self-harmed and that on a daily basis, I thought about suicide. Frequently, I was so overwhelmed by negative emotion that I could not function outside a work situation. When that environment was removed from me, some of my symptoms were suddenly more evident to my friends.

There is a perception of Mental Health problems as being something to be afraid of. I have begun to speak in public recently about mental health stigma and have been shocked that prejudice is found in all sorts of people from all walks of life. One of the responses is, 'But you can't have a complex mental health problem, you are not a violent person', which shows the need for real education about real people with real mental health issues. The fact is that you are more likely to be the victim of violent crime when you have a mental illness, than you are to be a perpetrator.

As with many taboo subjects, headlines and media mask the truth, and facts are neglected in exchange for selling more advertising, papers and programmes. I have found that this 'them' and 'us' gulf is best closed by speaking openly to people - when I'm well enough. I have also developed an upfront attitude to explaining why and where I can't cope with certain situations - 'I'm sorry, being around people today is just too painful for me.' I no longer do things out of deference to other people; I am learning that when I am struggling with my emotions I need to care for myself, in the same way that I would care for myself if I had 'flu. And instead of making something up I let them know that I am unwell, just as I would with 'flu. After all, both my BPD and the times when I have 'flu just tell me that I am a human being.

It is amazing that Mental Health is a subject that seems to be shrouded in mystery, something that is only discussed in hushed tones in corners. We may laugh at the older generations like my parents who refer to mental health problems as 'having trouble with your nerves'. But I'm not sure that modern attitudes are actually any more enlightened. They may have terms like depression and anxiety, but understanding has not developed any further than, 'Why don't you get out and about, get some fresh air and try to feel better!' Unless people actually HEAR what those of us with Mental Health issues say about how we are affected, then their understanding cannot develop any further. And if we are not engaging them in the conversation, then certainly no one is going to feel comfortable bringing up the subject.

The main thing I've found, as I've spoken to different groups locally, is that there are so many people out there who think they are the only ones who are struggling with mental health problems. The more we can talk to one another about the facts and reality of our illnesses and conditions, the more people will feel less isolated. Also, hopefully, the more people get to know individuals behind the diagnosis, the more they can see that actually it's not 'them' and 'us', but it's any one of us who can be affected by Mental Health issues.

Simon's Story

Living with a mental illness is draining, fractious and an all too often uncontrollable experience. An experience which is understood in depth by a small minority, but downplayed by a large majority. I can guarantee that anyone who has ever debated the topic "why is this happening to me?" with themselves will have come to no conclusion other than, "it simply isn't fair". That statement is true of so many people who suffered in silence, from Ernest Hemingway to Robin Williams – the unfair actuality is that the majority of friends I have made through mental health groups are the most creative, imaginative and intellective people I've ever known. They're fascinating, with talents that many would long to have themselves. Polly has offered us a fantastic opportunity to relay a message with this book so I don't want to write a piece which simply construes my issues to an audience of varying backgrounds and opinions. I want to use this chance to state exactly why mental health issues should be pivotal themes throughout society and then give the reasoning behind why stigmatisation of such a common problem remains so prevalent. During admissions to hospital and countless nights where sleep refused to arrive, I've been able to deeply evaluate these issues and I hope that every person who reads it will pick up on at least one point which challenges their thoughts - and it isn't intended to arrogate explicitly to those who have experienced some form of mental illness. It is completely my own opinion resulting from a range of experiences over the last seven years or so.

Most ailments we will encounter through our lives present visible indications, which more often than not lead to the exact problem being pinpointed, confirmed, then successfully treated. Looking for arrhythmia of the heart is found by doing an electrocardiogram. Abdominal problems can be found through the application of a computerised tomography scan. Infections can be discovered via blood tests. There are literally hundreds of diagnoses being made every single day by simple, non intrusive tests such as these. However, when it comes to abnormalities in the cognitive functions of the mind there are rarely any machines, scans, tests or screenings which lead to a precise, conclusive result - which for the patient is frustrating and doesn't give much hope for a sign that things will get better.

When facing someone downplaying the seriousness of my "off days" I simply compare the feelings inside my head as horrific and impacting on daily life with someone diagnosed with cancer. That is not a belittling or disparaging statement derogating the abominable experiences cancer patients face but merely a comparison to show that both are life-threatening diseases. Literally life-threatening. Statistically, in Britain, the greatest cause of death in males under thirty-five years old will be suicide – and it's fair to say that a number of these will have been tipped over the edge by the stigma of feeling ashamed at having a mental health problem. That's a higher percentage than any other illness within the same age range; add the fact that 16% of the teenagers inside that statistic will be facing homophobic stigmatisation and you begin to see how prevalent and dangerous an uneducated flippant comment can be to the vulnerable mind. This shock tactic often causes people to stop and reconsider their views on mental illness. Furthermore, the only reason I can find for the existence of these two diseases entering, then dwelling inside, the human body appears to be solely to break it or kill it then die – remember my opening paragraph: "it simply isn't fair". Perhaps when antagonists think about it in this way they will begin to take on board the seriousness of the issue. I know that unless certain areas of mental health treatment yield to science fairly rapidly it will during one of my "off days" be responsible for my death, just as a stage four cancer patient knows that will lead to theirs – that's how unequivocal the issue is and how it grinds anyone down to this level of bleakness after a while. However, through understanding and a little more acceptance from the population as a whole there is hope and opportunity to feel at ease with our day to day afflictions. Of course, I'm taking it to the extreme here but the sad fact is that so many victims do indeed end up in extreme situations so that's the angle I'll be coming from during this account.

I want to give a very brief overview of what it is like to live in partnership with a boisterous trespasser of the mind, just to set the scene for those who believe a good walk will bring about a miracle cure.

Imagine the most sombre, darkest moments you've ever encountered – no matter how trivial they may seem. Now with that feeling, conceptualise how you would feel if that was the most elated feeling you ever reached, but with the same emotion constantly nagging at your conscience, blowing the issue up to seem ten times as bad. In 2008, at the age of twenty-four, I had my first mental breakdown. To begin with, only a small part of me knew it was happening but I continued to function in my normal way of life. I was getting thinner, constantly confused, short tempered, having some very black thoughts, lackadaisical, slow, lethargic, pre-occupied, dirty through the lack of personal hygiene; but the subconscious, almost regimental, part of me was refusing to admit that anything was wrong. Having worked since I was sixteen and never had any health problems causing me to take time off work, it was as if my body was saying, "this is not an acceptable situation to be in" and continuing to drive me forwards, most probably based on the fact that mental health issues are not widely spoken about. If it was a common cold on the other hand I would have been straight to the pharmacy for some Lemsip (already a stark contrast between personal acceptance of varying ailments). Gradually, the inside of my head became one large numb bubble filled with smoke until my temples unrelentingly felt under pressure all day long. I made an appointment with the GP and can even remember my exact blank emotion as I sat on a radiator at work, staring out beyond reality, waiting for the time to pass until I was due to leave.

I was signed off with the all too common reason of "depression / anxiety" scrawled across the sick note. I have many issues with GPs using these two words as an umbrella to describe problems which are all unique to any one individual and strongly believe this adds fuel to the stigmatisation fire associated with mental health disorders; the reasoning for this I will come to shortly.

I walked in to that first appointment back in 2008 with an endogenous depression. There was no reason for it, no one trigger and no social distress, but I can guarantee that if the person before me had gone in feeling a little low because they were getting into debt they would have been given exactly the same sick note to give them time to sort things out. That's no reason to lack any compassion for that person but the two diagnoses, although in the same area, were at complete opposite ends of the spectrum and cannot really be classed as matching equivalents.

Fast forwarding from 2008 to the present, it's now June 2015 and during the year so far I've spent twice as much time hospitalised as I've spent at home. The years have been a series of ups and downs with various crises, interventions, therapies and combinations of medication mixed in. Desperately searching spiritually, medically, scientifically, even herbally for ways to ease the misery and get a grasp on the pendulum of mood as it swings from one extreme to the other. I've been lucky and always managed to stay one step ahead of my thoughts, clearly explaining to professionals how I feel but over the last few months I must admit it's begun to grind me down. I don't want anything, I don't have any ambition and I certainly don't enjoy anything to a level of contentedness. Choosing, then employing one of the many distraction techniques or actioning parts of a wellness plan really is as exhausting as a day's work and to carry on existing comes with a price, the price of living a "normal" life.

I could be sitting passively in the house gazing out through my eyes, seeing beyond my physical surroundings and looking into a cinematic loop of a finger drawing a figure of eight in sand. Over and over, repeatedly. No escape from it, no escape from the tightness I feel in my head, not being able to understand why I'm releasing this pent up angst by cutting my arms. It's like hosting a mystifying second being inside my body which feeds off the energy of my old self. In comes the psychosis, then the deeper and deeper depression until even the most positive of people would begin giving up. Almost all mental health issues cap the level of self worth and personal fulfilment to meaningless peaks unworthy of even acknowledging. In fact, my only claim to fame since experiencing these issues has been to single-handedly modify British Rail's timetable while I drained yet more tax payers' money to keep me safe. Another example of enforced mental burden resulting in guilt and mental scarring.

The uncertainty and inconsistency of my moods and emotions lead to simple things such as holding down a job, even one I love, to turn into the most demanding and wearying experience imaginable.

Hours spent in front of a mirror smearing various cosmetics into the bags under my eyes, which appear as a result of yet another insomnious night, telling a story to those looking at them. The energy involved in erecting a façade each morning to bluff my way through another day and appear well is utterly despairing after a while. Imagine having a job you enjoy but lack the mental capacity to actually carry it out without spiralling into maelstrom – remember my first paragraph, "it simply isn't fair". Even simple pleasures such as arranging to meet a friend in a week's time become a heavy worry rather than an enjoyment. I can't say whether I will feel too depressed or too anxious to get in the car and drive there. I can't even say I will have the mental capacity or motivation to string together a few sentences for a conversation on the phone. If I do make it I will undoubtedly turn up paranoid that the entire room will be looking at me, either because of my drawn and untidy appearance or the pungent odour coming from the preposterous amount of deodorant I have to use to mask the intense sweating that my medication causes.

Enjoyment and laughter become an experience of reminiscence, and even then the mind only allows them to be remembered when it gives me the capacity to do so. The incessant feeling that my brain is working flat-out processing thousands of thoughts every second is completely fatiguing. I have no idea what this brainpower is being used on and I find my concentration extremely poor as a result of it. The best description I can give is a feeling of constant preoccupation of the mind but with no result at the end of it. That is, if there ever is a brief end to it.

Anxiety is another issue which greatly burdens me – and no, it isn't just a feeling of nervous apprehension as a lot of audiences would describe it. True anxiety presents itself through a range of emotions; from guilt and self criticism to a real, acute fear which, when at its peak, will reach the point of looking over one's shoulder every few seconds or not being able to leave the house. It can get bad enough to cause nosebleeds, which is when I begin to despair. The moment a couple of steps are taken away from the front door every single window of surrounding buildings expands into large overbearing eyes which get bigger and bigger, closing in until eventually they would surely smother me had I not retreated back indoors covered in a dank film of sweat, breathless from the feeling of a lack of air in my lungs.

I'll end this sob story by summarising my mood over the last forty-eight hours. Yesterday the weather was pretty nice, I got out of bed, went outside into the garden with my camera and took some of the best, most creative, photos I've ever produced. I found inspiration from angles, colours and lighting which I'd previously never even thought of. I even had that old feeling of hot lead trickling into my stomach from the anticipation of seeing the photos on screen when I went back inside. Too good to be true. Sitting in the sun, camera in hand and waiting for a bee to land on a flower ready to take a close-up, a cloud so toxic and heavy descended upon me from the crown of my skull, creeping like thick oil down towards my feet until my whole body was deadened by its coverage. It was like I'd been sucked into the ground, unable to move and my mind became useless – the creativity and passion vanished as quickly as a shooting star. Numerous negative, destructive and self-criticising thoughts began to spin around in my mind, and the frustrating part is there was no noise, feeling or smell to trigger it. Back to my first paragraph, "it simply isn't fair". Towards the evening I began feeling a burning sensation down my forearms and thighs with a head so congested of empty thoughts I couldn't even remember the order of steps involved in making a cup of tea without focusing intensely. Wobbly calculations, weighing up whether I should call the Samaritans, Focus Line, Crisis Team or burden a friend, flickered like a candle blowing in the breeze. Of course I didn't phone anyone and simply lingered in a limbo of torment until it passed. I stayed awake as late into the night as possible, as normal, through fear of the nightmares and sleep paralysis that decide to play with me during the night. A hero of mine, the brilliantly unsettled Edgar Allan Poe, gorgeously summed this feeling up when he said, "sleep, those little slices of death - how I loathe them." After four hours of broken sleep I woke up feeling as low as a snake's belly, split seconds of fleeting thoughts wondering whether I should put my exit plan into action, desperately trying to do something that gives me an ounce of self value. Somehow I get through the day until tonight, as I write this, I feel better – I'm sat typing and I'm confident I'll finish it by the deadline. The hazy climate of my mind is smoggy and perturbed after the roller coaster of emotions condensed into just a few hours, but I'm alright. Tomorrow? Well let's wait and see.

So why is it so difficult to talk to people about mental health issues? Why do those who are affected worry themselves so much with how they appear or are perceived by others? What causes the guilty belief that these issues should be covered up? There are a number of reasons but the singular underlying constant is to prevent becoming a target to generalised stigmatic opinion and prejudgement from others. We've come a long way since the 16th century when someone with a mental illness may be deemed a witch and hunted down but there is still an air of snobbishness surrounding it. I myself have experienced a level of "polite disdainfulness" from branches of the family who see my suffering as a weakness rather than an unwanted burden. When asked how I am, they would rather dodge the question and answer in an uncommitted way than tell the exact truth. This makes it twice as difficult when I come face to face with people because I have to act exactly how they've been told I am. If only friends and family could begin to really understand, the whole experience would be so much better because it would open further doors of guidance and support.

Looking back in time I believe mental illness has been allowed to gain a certain air of mystique and taboo because the topic has been such an avoided concern amongst society for centuries. A chronological example: smallpox followed by polio followed by bronchitis followed by TB have all been austere medical issues but because they presented themselves with visual symptoms and affected classes from the rich to the poor they were researched and resolutions found. During this time mental health issues were always there running in parallel, but unpublicised, and anyone suffering was written off and thrown into an asylum. The shadows of that attitude, for some reason, continue to darken too many areas of society today - and had it not been for the fact that around one in four people now experience some type of mental grief I'm sure the practice would still be going on.

Wherever I've worked it's been common to hear people talk about one of their colleagues who was off with depression, and not in nice ways. The harsh level of non-acceptance in some examples was nothing more than a xenophobic orgy of verbal cruelty, it's no wonder that people don't like admitting to their issues when surrounded by such babyish conduct as this. Who would want to put themselves in a position to be spoken about like that? Accusing someone of "just wanting a bit of time off work" or "needing to man up" when they're probably at that very moment in time fighting terrible thoughts in their head, which these bigots will never experience, is so infuriating. We really shouldn't be made to feel incompatible with the normal regime of an office full of people. Remember the first paragraph? "It simply isn't fair". The ironic truth is that if the very same person was off work with their arm in plaster no one would even pass judgement.

This highlights the argument that if someone can actually see a plaster, wound, blood, splint or set of crutches, visually, the issue is accepted without question. But because mental health issues happen inside the head they are lesser thought of and open to abuse - regardless of the scars on one's arms or the bags under the eyes, the slurred speech or the silent presence. I can wholeheartedly say that the effects of medication, hospitalisation, therapies and personal degradation cannot be made up and no one would even attempt doing this for more than a month if they tried.

With new diagnoses being discovered it's imperative that we educate the nation as a whole, but especially unions, managers and colleagues at work, on the reality of mental health issues and how powerful stigmatic comments can be towards triggering self harm. Otherwise we run the risk of them knowing less and less about more and more, which I can already see beginning to happen. I've had managers who make no bones about telling me that I'm better off at work, keeping busy, mixing with people and taking my mind off things. What they don't realise is that there is a literal mental block on being able to get out of bed some days, let alone dressing and going in to work acting happy. It simply cannot be done; just as someone with a broken arm couldn't do their job as a bricklayer, someone with a mental health problem doesn't have the capacity to function.

I strongly believe that companies who have a policy of needing to be kept up to date with the situation of an employee when on long-term sick, need to re-evaluate how they go about obtaining this information. A string of phone calls and answerphone messages is the last thing I want to see on my phone. A sick note should qualify as their update on the situation, anything further is irrelevant. In the past I've been told to report in once a week, made to feel guilty at my lack of correspondence and much worse - which I won't mention here. What these employers don't understand is that by actually verbalising how I'm getting on, while at the same time trying to recover, it brings back a whole collection of memorability of experiences which I've tried so hard to forget, which is in itself enough to unsettle that "healed" part of the mind all over again. I've poured my energy into some workplaces but when my mental health takes a hit and I need time off I come to realise that I'm simply a row on a spreadsheet, which can be deleted and replaced with two clicks. This wouldn't happen with any other illness because a rough timescale of recovery can be estimated.

Leaving ignorance faced in the workplace to one side, I've noticed an increasing trend in celebrities blurting out controversial statements to gain personal publicity, which is completely unacceptable. I believe it should be equivalent of a hate crime to publicly derogate any mental health issue – with both the source and media which gives it the time of day equally punished. Examples are endless but a few months ago Katie Hopkins spent a few days writing a string of noxious bullying comments both in the Sun and on Twitter. I was in hospital at the time so it automatically hit a nerve with me but I watched intently as her followers actually rose during this period. Two such comments I remember were that "most depression is just genuine sadness at a social situation. Like being caught in torrential rain with a bag from Primark." and "....people with depression do not need a doctor and a bottle of something that rattles. They need a pair of running shoes and fresh air." How dare someone so uneducated on such matters use their position to spread hate in this manner! If 50% of her fans adopt her beliefs the impact on the work we carry out to cease this generic stigmatisation is instantly set back. What she is talking about is exogenous depression which yes, does exist, but is not anywhere near as aggressive as endogenous depression which I mentioned towards the beginning of this piece. Both are horrible to experience but to not make any division between the two and generalise in this manner is astonishingly moronic – especially coming from someone who suffers from epilepsy. Would anyone dare to belittle her when having an epileptic fit? I don't think so.

I can't let this area of stigma go without commenting on a very disappointing speech I listened to which included contributions from the author Will Self, someone whom I had a lot of respect for. He immediately set off on the wrong foot by stating that "a good brisk walk, talk with friend or heroin are just as effective as an SSRI - actually heroin is rather better". How many times have those of us with mental health issues been told this by someone, minus the heroin of course? I've had it preached to me by family, workmates, managers, and now people in the media who have no qualification to do so. A little later another small sentence during his speech, which almost slipped by unnoticed, was that SSRIs only work "because we are prescribed them by a doctor who says they work, we pay for them and we have faith in them, if you go home and begin to feel a bit funny you think, "oh I must be feeling better from my depression now"". He then went on to state that the reason these medications were nothing but placebos was backed up by the epic list of side effects each one warns of. If I came off my medications tomorrow I can categorically say that I would look differently, act differently and probably do something pretty stupid before long – and that isn't because I "believe" they work. I know they work. The dozens of combinations I've tried wouldn't have had any negative effects on me if they were all placebos – I would have simply risen higher and higher in mood until I reached a level of constant elation. He in fact trips himself up with these rather pompous comments because what he describes is the nocebo effect, that is the warning of possible side effects being enough for the brain to actually induce them physically, while talking about placebo feelings. If you're wondering what this has to do with stigma just think about the message it portrays, it's like saying mental health issues only affect valetudinarian individuals who can be "tricked" into feeling better with a pill containing nothing but sugar. I personally find this rather patronising.

The above is just an example of two semi-popular figures but there are scores more who feel the need to jump on the mental health bandwagon because they know that by referring to it in a stigmatic manner they will reap maximum attention of both those who suffer and those who don't. "Damnant quod non intellegunt" – they condemn what they do not understand.

Another reason why people find it difficult, nay refuse, to understand the issues we go through is described by TS Elliot when he said humankind "cannot bear too much reality". This is all too true in the case of mental health issues. Fear of not knowing what to do or how to respond to someone with such dark, bleak outlooks on life panics them into shutting their ears to it. Friends spoken to regularly slowly withdraw, politely but obviously, because they just don't know how to act around me – the few remaining ones are avoided through fear of scaring them away as well. Again, even a member of my own family hears the parts they want to but when something deemed strange, illogical or incomprehensible surfaces you can literally see it entering one ear and exiting the other because it cannot be processed.

It is only my own opinion but I don't think mental health issues will ever be conveyed as clearly and well defined as dementia or emphysema, for example, because psychology is not a science in the true sense of the word. And it never can be, as the areas researched are not accurately measurable in any reliable or valid sense. But with encouraging therapies and advances in the understanding of medications we can get through a day, albeit with the majority of our energy. I think the strongest lifeline I grab onto is "mindfulness" which appears to be taking the UK by storm at the moment. It should never be practised when hearing voices is prevalent but when out and about it's something that can be put into action without anyone around you even knowing. I use it in waiting rooms, noisy rooms – even when I went to vote in May. I would also promote the utilisation of any social groups held at nearby mental health hubs. Gradually these are spreading across the counties and even simply turning up and listening to others talk you realise that this isn't happening to you and you alone but also to a range of people from all different backgrounds and ages. No one understands you better than someone who has experienced it for themselves.

I hope I've managed to get a few points across – I can't seem to focus hard enough to say exactly what I wanted to but the gist is present. This has been the most demanding exercise I've done in a long while – it's taken me from the anxiety of whether I can accomplish it right through to the irritating frustration of not being able to remember the word I'm looking for. Again, jumping from this last paragraph to the very first one, remember, "it simply isn't fair", but it happens to those who least deserve it. Keep a strong faith – in anything, religiously, spiritually or simply in nature and when the stigma rises in front of you hold your head high and remember the traumatising experiences you've survived in the face of it all. We aren't victims of mental health problems any more, we're survivors. That's an accomplishment no other person can take away by a few verbal misconceptions.

Some Useful Online Resources

www.sane.org.uk

www.time-to-change.org.uk

www.mind.org.uk

www.rethink.org

www.youngminds.org.uk

www.mentalhealth.org.uk

www.maytree.org.uk

www.samaritans.org

www.mhchat.com

www.papyrus-uk.org

www.prevent-suicide.org.uk

www.psychcentral.com

www.depressionalliance.org

www.bpdworld.org

www.borderlinepersonalitydisorder.com

www.jigsawparenting.com

www.bipolaruk.org.uk

www.helpguide.org

www.together-uk.org

www.imaginementalhealth.org.uk

www.unitedresponse.org.uk

www.7cupsoftea.com

www.mentalhealthamerica.net

www.anxietyuk.org.uk

www.penumbra.org.uk

www.nopanic.org.uk

www.mentalhealthplatform.com

www.ingramcontent.com/pod-product-compliance
Lightning Source LLC
Chambersburg PA
CBHW051910170526
45168CB00001B/326